THE COMPLETE GUIDE TO
ASTROLOGICAL SELF-CARE

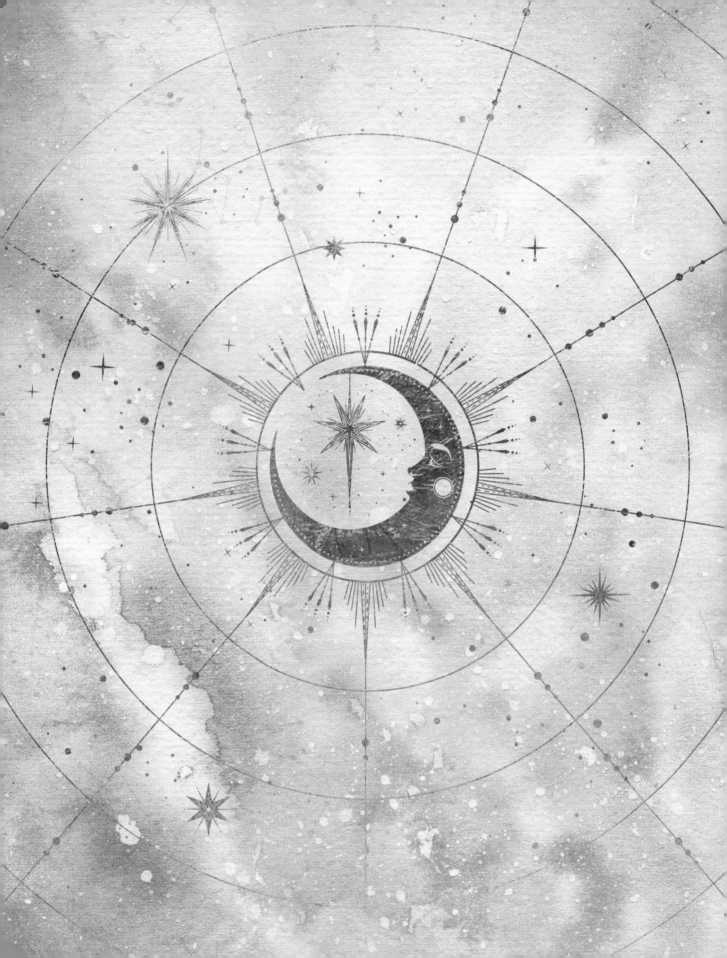

THE COMPLETE GUIDE TO
ASTROLOGICAL SELF-CARE

a holistic approach to wellness
for every sign in the zodiac

STEPHANIE GAILING

WELLFLEET
PRESS

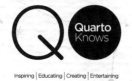

First published in 2021 by Wellfleet Press, an imprint of The Quarto Group
142 West 36th Street, 4th Floor, New York, NY 10018, USA
T (212) 779-4972 F (212) 779-6058 www.QuartoKnows.com

Wellfleet Press titles are also available at discount for retail, wholesale, promotional, and bulk purchase. For details, contact the Special Sales Manager by email at specialsales@quarto.com or by mail at The Quarto Group, Attn: Special Sales Manager, 100 Cummings Center Suite 265D, Beverly, MA 01915 USA.

10 9 8 7 6 5 4 3 2 1

ISBN: 978-1-57715-234-7

Library of Congress Cataloging-in-Publication Data available upon request.

Publisher: Rage Kindelsperger | Creative Director: Laura Drew | Managing Editor: Cara Donaldson
Senior Editor: John Foster | Cover Design: Sosha Davis | Interior Design: Kate Smith
Illustrations by Sosha Davis with the exception of pages 2, 12, 14, 17, 19, 22, 27, 34, 36, 48, 50, 64, 78, 90, 92, 104, 106, 120, 132, 134, 148, 160, 162, 176, 191, 192, 208, 210, 223, 244, 247, and 249.

Printed in China

CONTENTS

introduction

Years ago, to my delight, I discovered that there was a healing art that combined two of my greatest passions: astrology and health. Always looking for ways to inspire people to achieve their optimal well-being, I embarked on learning more about this approach, known as medical astrology.

With a long and legendary past, medical astrology is a healing art that views planetary placements as guiding stars to assess health and propose therapeutic treatments. It was documented by ancient Greek scholars, taught in medieval medical schools, and practiced by Renaissance physicians. In fact, up until the early twentieth century, many doctors employed its observations alongside other health-care methods. The study of the stars was so integral to the work of many healers that none other than the father of modern medicine, Hippocrates himself, was noted to have said, "He who does not understand astrology is not a doctor but a fool."

At the same time that I discovered medical astrology, I noticed that we were in the midst of a self-care revolution. People were realizing that the experience of health extended far beyond the absence of disease—that it also included their feeling their very best, in their mind, body, and spirit. We were becoming more active agents in our health care, on a quest for alternative approaches to feel more empowered, in control, and connected to nature and each other; to this aim, multitudes turned to natural and holistic therapies, practices, and remedies with more regularity in their pursuit of greater vitality.

Against this backdrop, I realized that the fundamental tenets of medical astrology could also be applied to the realm of wellness promotion. Rather than just focused on diagnosing and treating illness, it could be used as a framework to help us tap into more energy, reduce stress, gain greater awareness, and feel more aligned.

Recognizing the value of what I've come to call wellness astrology prompted me to write the pioneering book *Planetary Apothecary* over a decade ago as well as weave astrological self-care into my client and education work, helping people the world over to access a stellar approach to well-being. Over time, I have come to appreciate that this healing art has even more benefits than I initially realized; in addition to our planetary profile helping us personalize our self-care regimen, a wellness-astrology orientation can gift us a universe of other rewards. Since astrology is a tool that helps us understand the different phases of life we pass through, it also gives us a method to identify and address our wellness needs at different life stages. And, because it offers us a way to further understand the *kairos*, the opportunity inherent within different moments (see page 9), we can see how the paths of the planets can help inform the paths we can take at different periods to bolster our sense of vibrancy. *The Complete Guide to Astrological Self-Care* addresses all of these facets, providing you with a timeless resource that will help you access a galaxy of salutary knowledge.

At this point, you may be wondering: What is the connection between astrology and health? At the heart of medical astrology is the axiom "as above, so below," reflecting the long-held belief in the connection between the celestial bodies and our own bodies. Throughout history, the zodiac signs and their ruling planets have been associated with various body parts,

A Manual for Stellar Self-Care

Part I of this book features sections for each of the twelve zodiac signs, each including details on scores of wellness strategies that are particularly aligned with their unique temperaments and tendencies. And while you may want to focus on honing in on those highlighted for your personal astrology profile, don't limit yourself to just reading those sections. That's because with the spectrum of wellness suggestions featured in *The Complete Guide to Astrological Self-Care*, it can serve as a veritable guidebook to support your well-being and that of your family and friends.

Awareness as Self-Care

Awareness can be an antidote to stress. If we're caught off guard by an experience, we may feel rattled and filled with disquietude. Yet, if we're cognizant that a certain moment in time will bring with it certain opportunities and/or challenges, we can then view experiences that unfold through this lens. This not only gives us the ability to better understand what may be occurring but also approach situations more calmly. It's for this reason that being aware of the unique invitations that different moments yield—whether the Stellar Life Stages (pages 189–193), the New and Full Moons (pages 207–209), or the Planetary Retrogrades (pages 237–238) —can be an important step in finding ways to feel a greater sense of well-being. As we know, knowledge is power, and in this case a powerful self-care strategy.

physiological functions, and emotional tendencies. The signs and planets have also been accorded signature correspondences with different members of the plant, mineral, and animal kingdoms. Additionally, knowing which ones are playing a starring role in the sky at any time can help us zero in on the invitations that different moments offer, allowing us to orient in ways that minimize stress and optimize well-being.

What You'll Discover in This Book

The Complete Guide to Astrological Self-Care covers a gamut of wellness astrology topics, organized into four parts:

PART 1: ZODIAC SIGNS

In the first part, you'll find twelve sections—one dedicated to each of the zodiac signs. Each section includes individualized wellness profiles as well as holistic health approaches targeted for each unique astrological personality.

PART 2: STELLAR LIFE STAGES

In the second part, you'll discover a cosmic road map that will help you navigate your wellness needs throughout life, from your twenties through your eighties. You'll learn about the invitations of different phases of life as well as the self-care strategies that may help you bolster your vitality.

PART 3: THE MOONS

Here you'll discover how to align your well-being with the lunar cycle. You'll learn about the different Moon phases as well as access details on the wellness opportunities and challenges offered by the twenty-four different New Moons and Full Moons we experience each year.

PART 4: PLANETARY RETROGRADES

These sections demystify the retrograde cycles of Mercury, Venus, and Mars, showing you how you can make the most of these times. You'll access perspectives and self-care strategies that can help you feel more connected and aligned.

In addition to providing you with a modern approach to an ancient healing art, *The Complete Guide to Astrological Self-Care* is replete with details on hundreds of natural remedies and holistic strategies, making it a reference guide you can turn to time and again. Through it you will see that while the planets are far away, with the insights we can glean from them thanks to astrology, wellness is actually much closer than we think.

The Time for Self-Care: Chronos and Kairos

In ancient Greece, there were two terms used when referring to time: *chronos* and *kairos*. Chronos signifies the quantity of time. For example, if you're noting that something will happen in a minute, a week, or a year, you're speaking of chronos. Alternatively, kairos refers to the quality inherent in distinct moments in time, the possibilities that are embedded within those moments. When we sense that different epochs in history, periods in our lives, or even instances throughout our day have their own unique themes, patterns, and qualities that are quite distinct than others, it's the kairos that we're tapping into. By translating the archetypal potentials of planetary placements and alignments occurring at different moments, astrology can help us decipher the kairos. It gives us awareness as to the opportunities and challenges intrinsic in different periods, and with that we can turn to astrology for a wealth of understanding, including how to curate a stellar approach to self-care.

PART I:

zodiac
signs

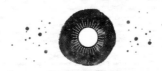

THE SIGNS OF SELF-CARE

How do you navigate the maze of self-care options available to curate a wellness strategy that mirrors your individual needs? A great place to start is with your astrology chart. Throughout history, medical astrologers would view personal planetary profiles as repositories of wellness wisdom: they used astrology charts to assess their clients' constitutions, determine the best remedies and therapies for them, suggest timing of proposed treatments, and evaluate underlying psycho-emotional patterns that might keep them from optimal health.

Yet, you don't need to consult with a medical astrologer to enjoy some of the benefits that this healing art offers. As every zodiac sign paints a unique portrait of the way we define, express, and relate to health, even knowing the very basics of your astrology chart can offer you stellar access to well-being.

What do I mean by basics? Even if you just know your Sun sign, you can connect to a wealth of knowledge that can help you take your self-care strategies to the next level. And if you know your Moon and Ascendant signs—which you can readily access if you know the time you were born—you can further understand the nuances of your temperament and tendencies so that you can better meet your needs and take care of yourself.

The following twelve sections go into details about the cosmic health profiles associated with each zodiac sign. Reading the section associated with your Sun sign—as well as your Moon and Ascendant signs if you know them—will help you better recognize your unique strengths and stressors, and the lifestyle strategies and remedies that can support and sustain your well-being.

Your Sun, Moon, and Ascendant Signs

SUN SIGN

When most people think about their astrology profile, they focus upon their Sun sign (what you answer when someone asks, "What's your sign?"). As the Sun represents your vitality and the essence of who you are, the sign in which it resides can tell you a lot about your individual wellness profile. Therefore, reading your Sun sign section is the first step in designing a stellar self-care approach.

Our Sun signs are the easiest to determine as all they require is knowing our birthday. If you don't already know your Sun sign, look below to discover it. Yet note that each year the Sun may change signs a day or after the ones noted.

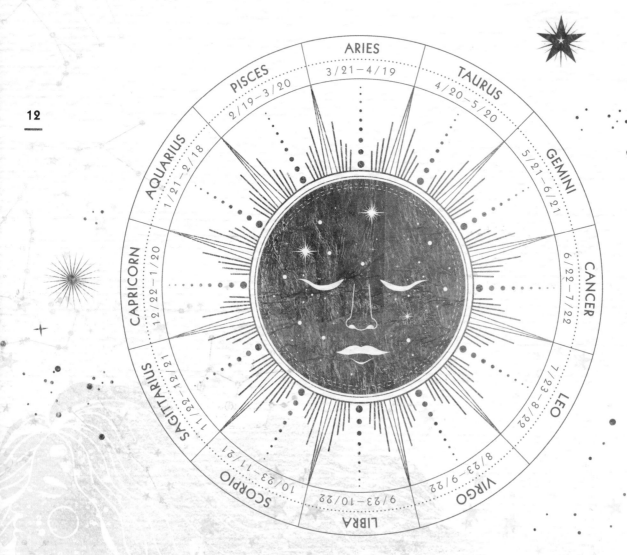

Therefore, if your birthday is on the cusp, you'll want to calculate your chart to determine what Sun sign you are. You can readily do so using one of the websites listed in the Resources section (page 252) or by consulting with a professional astrologer.

MOON SIGN

Your Moon sign embodies your emotional being. Learning more about it can help you better learn how to nourish yourself, connect to your feelings, and understand how to feel more at home in your body and your life. Reading the section on your Moon sign will have you more attuned to ways to take the best care of yourself and provide you with clues as to the health-care approach you may find particularly nurturing, both for your physical health and emotional well-being.

ASCENDANT (OR RISING) SIGN

The Ascendant—also referred to as the Rising Sign—is a key feature of your astrology chart that symbolizes the way in which you present yourself to the world. It represents how you engage with the environment and navigate your life. Additionally, it's thought to describe characteristics of our physical body, making it a noteworthy signifier of health. Therefore, exploring the section on your Ascendant sign can help you further recognize steps you can take to curate your personalized self-care strategies and fortify your well-being.

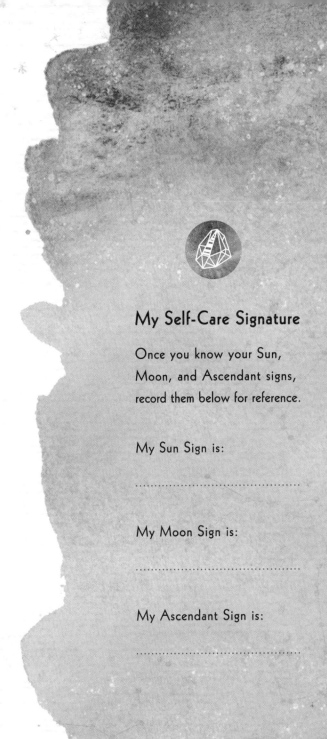

My Self-Care Signature

Once you know your Sun, Moon, and Ascendant signs, record them below for reference.

My Sun Sign is:

....

My Moon Sign is:

....

My Ascendant Sign is:

....

If you don't already know your Moon and Ascendant signs, you can discover them through casting your chart online or having an astrologer do it for you. (See page 252 for the resources to do so.) As you explore the sections on your Sun, Moon, and Ascendant signs, see which suggestions from each most deeply resonate with you, something that may change during different times in your life. Some people have the Sun, Moon, and Ascendant in different signs while others may find that there's a sign in which two—or even three—of them reside. If the latter's the case for you, it means that that sign plays an even more important role in reflecting who you are, and what your health and wellness needs may be.

Symbols, Planetary Rulers, Elements, and Modalities

One of the ways that we can gain more understanding as to the proclivities and personalities associated with each zodiac sign is by learning about its symbol, planetary ruler, element, and modality. This information is included in the first page of each of the following twelve sections. So that you can further understand the key insights they offer, here is some background information. On page 16, you'll find an overview chart; not only will this help you see each sign's attributes at a glance, but you'll be able to see qualities shared by different signs.

SYMBOLS

Each of the twelve zodiac signs has a symbol with which it is associated. Recognizing the characteristics the symbol expresses helps us further connect to the sign, aiding us in understanding what it represents. Additionally, by reviewing what meaning a symbol held throughout mythological and cultural traditions, we can further perceive attributes accorded with the zodiac sign.

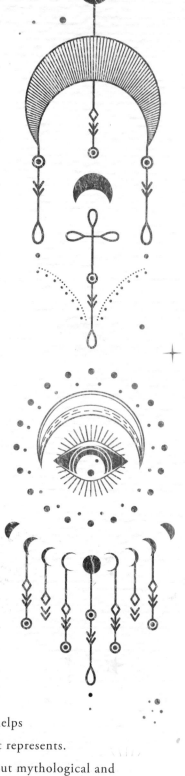

All of the twelve signs are represented by either a human or animal figure, except for one (Libra, the symbol for which is a scale).

PLANETARY RULERS

Since ancient times, each sign was granted a connection with a planet that was visible in the night sky, known as its classical planetary ruler. Not only is each planet said to have more strength when it's in the sign that it rules, but there is an alliance that exists between the planets and the signs that they govern. Therefore, when you examine the characteristics of the celestial bodies themselves, as well as the archetypal qualities that correspond with their eponymous mythic deities, you can glean a lot about the signs with which they are associated. After the telescope was invented, and Uranus, Neptune, and Pluto were discovered, each of these planets was assigned governance over a sign as well; they are referred to as their modern planetary ruler. Therefore, you'll notice that some signs have one planetary ruler while others have two.

ELEMENTS

Since antiquity, and in numerous wisdom traditions throughout the world, the universe has been seen as composed of elements, the presence of which is used to explain and describe the nature of matter. As a way to further describe the meaning of the twelve astrological signs, each has come to be associated with one of the four classical elements: fire, earth, air, and water. There are three zodiac signs associated with each of the elements. By knowing the nature of the element with which a zodiac sign is associated, we can further understand its characteristics and temperament, which can provide important insights that allow us to know ourselves—and our wellness needs—better.

MODALITIES

Another way that astrological signs are organized is by their modality—also referred to as states or qualities—of which there are three: cardinal, fixed, and mutable. There are four zodiac signs associated with each of the modalities. The modalities express aspects of the creation cycle: when something emerges (cardinal), when it solidifies into form (fixed), and when it goes through the process of change and reformation (mutable). The modality associated with each sign gives us further insight into its hallmark characteristics and some of its personality traits.

SIGN	PLANETARY RULER	ELEMENT	MODALITY
ARIES	MARS	FIRE	CARDINAL
TAURUS	VENUS	EARTH	FIXED
GEMINI	MERCURY	AIR	MUTABLE
CANCER	MOON	WATER	CARDINAL
LEO	SUN	FIRE	FIXED
VIRGO	MERCURY	EARTH	MUTABLE
LIBRA	VENUS	AIR	CARDINAL
SCORPIO	MARS* PLUTO**	WATER	FIXED
SAGITTARIUS	JUPITER	FIRE	MUTABLE
CAPRICORN	SATURN	EARTH	CARDINAL
AQUARIUS	SATURN* URANUS**	AIR	FIXED
PISCES	JUPITER* NEPTUNE**	WATER	MUTABLE

For signs that have two planets associated with it, * represents its classical ruler and ** its modern-day ruler

What's Featured in Each Zodiac Sign Section

Every section opens by exploring the fundamentals of that particular zodiac sign. In addition to general characteristics, it also covers information about its symbol, planetary ruler, element, and modality (see opposite page), all of which can provide further understanding of your unique astrological temperament. It also features the following eleven sections:

PERSONAL HEALTH PROFILE

Discover the attitudes that shape your sign's approach to wellness. Here you'll get a glimpse into the innate tendencies and habits that affect your sign's unique well-being and the arenas of self-care to which you may be especially attracted.

AREAS OF HEALTH FOCUS

Different parts of the body are associated with each of the twelve signs, as are different personality propensities that influence our ability to connect to optimal health. These may be inherent areas of vulnerability, but when attended to, they can become realms of strength.

HEALTHY EATING TIPS

Natives of each sign have different personalities, which can lead to dietary habits that either support or stand in the way of optimal health. This section provides healthy eating tips that are geared toward your unique temperament and that can help you boost overall healthfulness.

HEALTH-SUPPORTING FOODS

Here you'll learn about foods that have a special affinity for each sign, whether because of a traditional association or because they address concerns specific to a unique astrological profile.

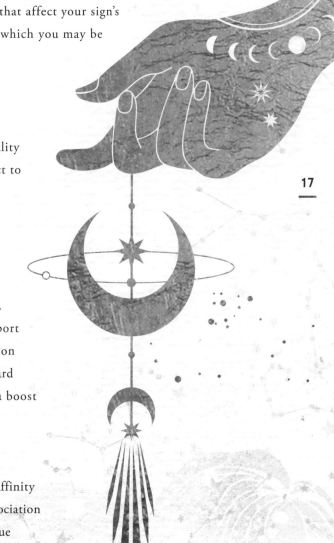

Homeopathics

Homeopathic remedies are extremely diluted forms of the natural substance from which they are made. Mint and coffee can counteract the effectiveness of homeopathics, so avoid them for several hours before and after taking these remedies. Like with the other natural remedies, homeopathics can be found in natural food stores or holistic pharmacies or through health-care practitioners.

WELLNESS THERAPIES

Wellness therapies include activities provided by trained practitioners, which you can enjoy at a spa or health clinic; some can also be adapted to be done at home. Each of these natural health treatments has its own style and benefits; as such, some are better matched to the personalities and health characteristics of different signs.

RELAXATION PRACTICES

Distinct from wellness therapies, relaxation practices are more self-directed activities that you can do on your own. As each fulfills a different need and is attuned to a distinct constitution, certain ones are more in sync with particular zodiac signs.

NATURAL REMEDIES

There are a variety of natural remedies—whether dietary supplements, herbs, or homeopathics—that can offer benefit for zodiac-related wellness concerns. Additionally, the planets and signs have long-established correspondences with the many plants and nutrients that comprise different natural remedies.

ESSENTIAL OILS

Aromatherapy is a healing art that uses essential oils—the fragrant essences of plants—to foster well-being. Essential oils are distilled from the flowers, fruits, leaves,

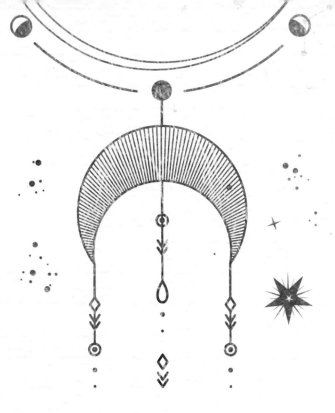

and wood of many different botanicals. With their distinctive qualities, as well as the astrological correspondence that exists between plants and planets, it makes sense that certain scents are especially suited for different signs.

FLOWER ESSENCES

These natural elixirs, made from flower-infused water, work energetically to restore mental and emotional balance. Various flower essences accord with distinct psycho-emotional constitutions and, as such, address the unique tendencies associated with each of the zodiac profiles.

YOGA POSES

Yoga provides a holistic approach to exercise that increases physical strength and

Using Essential Oils

There are a variety of ways you can incorporate essential oils into your self-care regimen. You can use them in an aromatherapy diffuser to fragrance a room; small ones that plug into a car's lighter can make a great alternative to synthetic air fresheners. You can mix several drops in a carrier base—such as almond, avocado, or jojoba—and use as a massage oil or moisturizer. Adding some to a mister bottle filled with water can create a facial toner or environmental room spray. And, of course, you can smell the fragrances right from their bottles any time you want to enjoy their beautiful scents.

Using Flower Essences

You can use flower essences either orally or topically. For the former, the recommended dosage is usually four drops of each four times a day. You can take them straight from the container, add them to 1 cup (250 ml) of water, or put them in a glass dropper bottle filled with water. You can use them topically by placing them on your skin or adding them to a bath, or putting four drops of each in a mister bottle that contains water (and an essential oil, if you'd like) and spritzing yourself or your environment several times a day. While multiple flower essences can be used in a blend, many practitioners suggest not including more than five at once. Flower essences can be found in natural food stores and holistic pharmacies.

flexibility while calming the mind and inspiring the spirit. While there are hundreds of yoga poses (also known as *asanas*) that can benefit general well-being, certain poses target particular body parts or health concerns, and therefore may be more aligned with specific astrological signs.

INSPIRING SLEEP

Getting good sleep is an inherent facet of stellar self-care. Given that all twelve signs have unique temperaments, each one may benefit from different slumber-inspiring tips.

As you journey through the next twelve sections, you'll not only explore which foods, natural remedies, and activities are most supportive of each sign but also *why* they are beneficial. Really understanding your individual needs, both physical and emotional, is vital to living a healthy and balanced life. If you know what makes you tick, it follows that you will have an easier time integrating these habits and choices into your routine. After all, health is not just something measured by the absence of illness or discomfort but by the vitality that is experienced when you live in sync with your true nature.

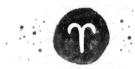

ARIES

CHARACTERISTICS

Assertive, brave, carefree, direct, energetic, enterprising, hot-tempered, impatient, impulsive, individualistic, pioneering, willful.

SYMBOL

The Ram, an animal known for its strength, will, and competitive nature. In mythological and cultural traditions, the Ram is a symbol of power, new beginnings, and renewal.

PLANETARY RULER

Mars, often called the "Red Planet" in reference to its color. Mars was the Roman god of war and fertility, known for his ability to fight, defend, and protect. His counterpart in Greek mythology was Ares. In astrology, Mars represents desire, courage, self-initiation, and a call to action.

ELEMENT

Fire, characterized by the dynamic energy of inspiration, enthusiasm, and passion. It is transformative, kinetic, and action oriented. Movement, spontaneity, and tapping into their imagination energizes fire signs while slowness, stagnancy, and a sense of limitation may deplete their vitality.

MODALITY

Cardinal, which loves beginnings and the first stage of a creative project. Cardinal signs are motivated, ambitious, and enterprising. They encounter stress when things are not fresh and new.

Personal Health Profile

Aries are blessed with great vitality. After all, yours is the first sign of the zodiac, reflecting the burgeoning of new life. Your tremendous energy reserves and fiery spirit make you well poised for experiencing abundant health and longevity.

When you do get sick, you take it seriously and, like a true Ram, face the situation head-on. For an Aries, illness becomes yet another thing to conquer, eliciting your inner warrior. And conquer it you must, since you want to return quickly to the playing field of life. Sitting on the sidelines is unbearable for your feisty spirit.

While assertive Aries are often armed with clear strategies to reach their wellness goals, they are sometimes short on the patience required to see them through. As with all you take on, you like to see immediate results. If you don't get that near-instant gratification from your well-intentioned actions, you may feel tempted to abandon even your best-laid plans.

One way to stay the course is to set smaller, easier-to-accomplish goals. For example, don't establish a hard-to-achieve target of losing 4 pounds (2 kg) in one week; instead, shoot for 1 to 2 pounds (.5 to 1 kg), a mark that you can more readily accomplish week after week. This strategy for achieving your wellness goals will honor your action-oriented nature while helping to temper your impatience, bringing optimal health more immediately within your grasp.

As Aries are pioneers, you will likely try many wellness activities and natural remedies before others have even heard of them. The ones that best serve you are those that honor your active nature. Sitting passively is not for you, as you want to be involved and engaged. Channeling your energy into an exercise program can be one way to champion your well-being.

When a health issue calls for some outside assistance, it's important to find a practitioner who involves you directly in decision making; after all, just as in many areas of your life, it's important for you to feel like you are playing an active role in staking your claim. Because, to an Aries, there's no point in not getting to the point, your ideal medical specialists are straightforward communicators who display candor and honesty, qualities that the Ram appreciates.

Areas of Health Focus

The parts of the body associated with Aries include:

- The **head** and **brain**, which control physical and mental activities
- The **muscular system**, which gives you strength
- The **blood**, which carries energizing oxygen to the muscles and all of the body's organs
- The **adrenal glands**, which govern the stress response and the fight-or-flight mechanism

Your Aries pioneering spirit, strong will, and formidable instincts are some of the resources you can use when facing any health challenge.

STAY AHEAD OF HEADACHES

As Aries rules the head and brain, accumulated stress may take root there, making you vulnerable to headaches, some powerful enough to stop you right in your tracks. Taking time to relax, in whatever ways best suit your on-the-go nature, is important when you get a headache (and for preventing them in the first place). Additionally, keep tabs on your diet to see if any particular foods lead to a throbbing noggin; for example, many migraine sufferers are sensitive to aged cheese, sour cream, red wine, and chocolate. And don't forget to keep your water intake flowing throughout your busy day, as dehydration is a leading cause of headaches.

PREVENT STRAINS AND SPRAINS

Your ruling planet, Mars, governs the muscular system, which is integral to all things Aries, including movement and action. To protect your muscles, try to override your impetuous instincts long enough to stretch and warm up before you dive into your exercise routine. If you find that you're prone to muscle cramps, consider increasing your intake of magnesium-rich foods such as green vegetables, seeds, and fish. With Aries ruling the head, you may be prone to carrying some of the stress in your facial and jaw muscles; when you go for a massage, make sure the therapist works on this area to release any pent-up tension. And as you zip from one activity to the next, be careful to avoid accidental mishaps that can result in strains, sprains, and bruises.

SUPPORT YOUR ADRENAL GLANDS

Aries are always on alert, ready to respond to the situation at hand without even batting an eye. Yet, if your nervous system is constantly geared up for battle, it may tax your energy reserves, depleting your adrenal glands and impacting your long-term ability to effectively respond to stress. Luckily, you can be proactive on the nutrition front and boost your adrenals by curbing excess caffeine intake and ensuring your diet features adequate amounts of foods rich in vitamin B5, such as yogurt, sunflower seeds, mushrooms, and corn. Consider adaptogenic herbs (a class of herbs that enhance the body's resistance to stress), such as eleuthero, ashwagandha, and/or rhodiola rosea, which are thought to be supportive of the body's stress response.

REST AND RECUPERATE

Aries are on the go from the get-go. Your pep and verve get you moving and keep you moving long after others have called it a day. Your energetic nature knows no bounds, which can be a boon when you're healthy and yet a challenge when you're not. Since you're used to being on the move, taking the time to rest and recuperate is not necessarily your forte. Yet, remember that doing so is often the best strategy to help you quickly shore up your energy reserves, putting you back on the fast track to vibrant health with all of your vitality in tow.

Healthy Eating Tips

While Aries are often on the run, it's important to take the time to stop (even for a moment) to nourish yourself with health-promoting foods that can kindle your energy and vitality.

TAKE TIME TO EAT BREAKFAST

Out of the gate running, Aries like to avoid obstacles that seem to slow them down, with one such perceived barrier to getting the day under way being eating breakfast. Yet it's no understatement that breakfast can be the most important meal of the day, and even a quick one can provide you with the lasting energy you need to power through your bustling schedule. Ideas for a quick and energizing morning meal include a hard-boiled egg, whole-wheat crackers and almond butter, or muesli mixed with nuts and dried fruit. If you don't have time to eat at home, you can always brown bag it to work or school.

COOL IT

Fire-sign Aries often crave foods that are spicy and hot. While piquant foods can fan your inner flames, an overabundance of heat, according to Ayurvedic medicine (a healthcare system that originated in India that is gaining popularity across the West today), may cause rashes and irritability. When it comes to spicy foods, the key is moderation—not a concept that comes easily to Aries, but one that is important to practice. If you want to balance out the heat, enjoy cooling foods such as sweet fruit, basmati rice, sprouts, and watery vegetables (including lettuce and cucumbers). In Ayurvedic nutrition, poultry is considered more cooling than red meat; the latter is thought to aggravate the fiery constitution to which an Aries may be prone. And, if you feel overheated between meals, mint tea or filtered water can help cool you down.

IRON OUT YOUR DIET

Aries governs the blood as well as the mineral iron. For optimal health, you'll want to make sure your diet includes adequate supplies of this nutrient, which functions to oxygenate your blood and muscles. While meat is a ready source of iron, you can also get your fix of this important mineral via a cornucopia of plant-based foods. Vegetarian foods that will help you meet your iron goals include spinach, chard, pumpkin seeds, beans, and lentils. If you want a sweetener that will energize you with its iron content, try blackstrap molasses.

Health-Supporting Foods

Fruits, vegetables, sprouts, and other foods that capture the energy of spring can help your vitality bloom. Foods associated with your planetary ruler, Mars, may also be health-promoting to an Aries' diet.

SPROUTS

Just like the sign of Aries, sprouts represent the initial stages of growth, when all that can exist first bursts onto the scene, declaring itself to the world. Sprouts contain concentrated amounts of nutrients and contribute to a sense of well-being. In addition to popular alfalfa sprouts, look for those made from mung beans and lentils as well as broccoli, sunflower, and radish seeds. A great way to enjoy your favorite sprouts is to top a sandwich or green salad with them. Also, look for bread made from sprouted grains. Not only does sprouted bread taste great, but many people claim that it is easier to digest.

GARLIC

Garlic has long been associated with your planetary ruler, Mars. Like the mythic Mars, garlic is a warrior; its ability to fight off bacteria and viruses has been well documented. It is also very good for circulatory health, reducing cholesterol and triglyceride levels as well as platelet stickiness. No matter what cuisine you favor, you're bound to find recipes that include garlic, as it is a prized ingredient in many cultures. As studies have found raw garlic to provide some unique health benefits compared to its cooked counterpart, be sure to include it in your diet; adding raw garlic to salad dressings, guacamole, and salsas can amplify their flavor, and your well-being.

RED FOODS

Red is associated with Aries: it's the color of your element, fire, as well as the brilliant hue that emanates from Mars. So why not enjoy an arsenal of nutrient-rich red foods? For example, beets are rich in appetite-satisfying fiber, tomatoes are filled with heart-healthy lycopene, and cayenne peppers contain pain-relieving capsaicin. You can roast whole beets in the oven for a deliciously sweet side dish or try a twist on traditional hummus by including them in the recipe. Since fat increases lycopene absorption, to enhance the nutrient power of tomatoes, add some extra virgin olive oil to recipes that feature them. And, make salsa even redder by adding some cayenne pepper (but only a pinch so you don't overheat).

Wellness Therapies

While it may be challenging for an Aries to stop long enough to enjoy a wellness therapy, doing so every now and again can be very valuable to your health.

SHIRODHARA

Shirodhara is an Ayurvedic healing treatment focused on the Aries-ruled head. Warm herb-infused sesame oil is gently poured onto the center of your forehead. The slow-flowing oil cascades onto your scalp and neck, which then receive an invigorating massage. Shirodhara is also said to aid in relaxation and foster mental clarity, possibly through its ability to increase the brain's alpha waves, which is associated with greater serenity. As a therapy, it's been used to treat headaches, sinusitis, and allergies. While shirodhara is performed in many spas and the offices of Ayurvedic health-care practitioners, with the help of a friend, you can do a modified shirodhara treatment at home.

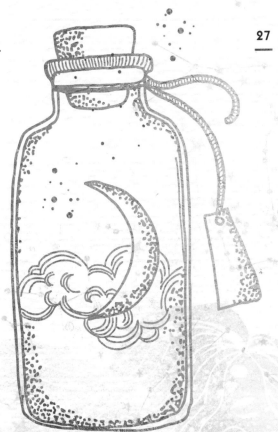

CRANIOSACRAL THERAPY

Another treatment that focuses on the Aries-ruled head is craniosacral therapy. The term *craniosacral* refers to the cranium (the head) and the sacrum (the bone in the lower back). This very gentle form of bodywork relieves tension and enhances the circulation of cerebrospinal fluid. A good portion of a craniosacral session involves the practitioner cradling and gently rocking your head, working to balance cranial rhythms and lightly adjusting the cranial bones. Reported benefits of this relaxing therapy include the reduction of chronic headaches and mental stress, and the relief of neck and back pain. As one of the more gentle treatments, it is a common form of bodywork used on children.

MOXIBUSTION

Akin to acupuncture (see page 167), and sometimes used in combination with it, moxibustion is a treatment widely used in traditional Asian medicine to address a wide range of health imbalances. Yet unlike acupuncture, moxibustion is noninvasive, using the power of Aries' heat to induce healing. Practitioners either hold a stick of burning dried moxa (mugwort herb) above a target spot or place a heated kernel of it directly on the skin, oftentimes on top of a slice of Aries-ruled ginger. Moxibustion is said to stimulate the circulation of blood as well as the vital energy known as *chi*. Warming an inserted needle with a moxa stick is said to further its ability to stimulate energy flow.

 # Relaxation Practices

Engaging in activities that give your fiery spirit a vehicle for expression can be very grounding and calming to an Aries.

WALKING MEDITATION

If the idea of meditation intrigues you but your active spirit finds the thought of sitting still for a spell of time an unattractive prospect, walking meditation may be right up your alley. During this relaxation exercise, you focus your attention on your breath and/or a mantra while meandering in a predetermined path, whether around your neighborhood or your home. As in other forms of meditation, it's normal if thoughts come into your mind. Notice them and then let them pass, returning your attention to your breath or mantra. While some people find silence golden during this practice, others find it easier to concentrate while listening to a guided meditation.

MARTIAL ARTS

Participating in one of the many martial arts practices will help you get in touch with your inner warrior while providing a fun (and intense) workout. The martial arts are an effective way to get in shape, relieve stress, and gain the confidence that comes from knowing how to defend yourself. Since you can choose from a variety of traditions—including tae kwon do, aikido, kendo, and judo—you're sure to find one that suits your personal style. Many studios (known as dojos) will allow you to observe classes, so you can see whether the particular practice methods are of interest to you before signing up. As some dojos offer online classes, you can also practice martial arts at home.

FIERY CRAFTS

As Aries are blessed with creativity, and since the element of fire is associated with your sign, why not channel your artistic energy by crafting objects using the power of flame? Take a glassblowing class and transform molten glass into radiant objects of beauty. If making jewelry is of more interest, consider metalworking. As your sign is associated with iron, you could also try your hand at blacksmithing. Art schools and community colleges may be your best bets for learning these crafts. Survey courses will introduce you to a range of techniques so you can see which one is the most appealing.

 # Natural Remedies

Supplements, herbs, and homeopathics can be a first-line defense against many everyday health challenges.

IRON SUPPLEMENTS

Iron is a mineral that keeps the Aries-ruled blood oxygenated. If you suspect your diet isn't providing you with enough, consider taking some as a dietary supplement. While iron supplements come in a variety of forms, you might want to avoid ferrous sulfate as some people find it causes nausea and constipation. Instead, consider easy-to-assimilate chelated types, which aren't known for gastrointestinal side effects. If you want iron in a non-pill form, look for a liquid supplement made from fruits, vegetables, and herbs. While too little iron is problematic, so is too much; if you supplement with this nutrient, have your physician regularly monitor your iron levels.

HOMEOPATHIC ARNICA (*ARNICA MONTANA*)

Homeopathic arnica is a very useful addition to an Aries' first-aid kit. Right after an injury occurs, especially a muscular strain or sprain, take arnica to reduce any associated pain and swelling. It's also great for soothing bruises and relieving any muscle soreness caused by overexertion. And, if you're scheduled for dental work, arnica's anti-inflammatory properties may be just what the doctor ordered. In addition to arnica pills, this homeopathic remedy is available as an ointment or gel for topical applications. Mint and coffee can counteract the effectiveness of homeopathic remedies, so avoid them for several hours before and after taking arnica.

NETTLE (*URTICA DIOICA*)

Nettle is one of the main herbal remedies used for hay fever, a reaction to the pollen released by flowers and trees in bloom. While stumbling onto a patch of stinging nettle can cause a rash that's fiery hot, with its poisonous bristles deactivated—by cooking, drying, or crushing—this herb's amazing health-promoting compounds are able to shine. You can find nettle available in capsule or liquid tincture form. You can also enjoy fresh or dried nettle leaves, boiled or steamed in soups and other dishes, or enjoyed as a tea.

 ## Essential Oils

Aromatherapy can provide the Aries warrior with a fragrant way to defend their well-being that doesn't require much of a time commitment.

GINGER (*ZINGIBER OFFICINALE*)

With its name derived from the Sanskrit word for "horn," ginger essential oil may be well suited for Rams and their wellness needs. It is an effective oil for muscle aches due to overexertion during exercise. And if you're prone to motion sickness, ginger essential oil may do the trick, as it is one of the best steadying remedies around. In addition, its warming fragrance inspires passion, and you can use it if you ever need to stoke your libidinal fire. When you feel under the weather, add ginger and lemon juice to a bath for a pick-me-up. You can also use ginger-scented massage oil as a healing salve for sore muscles. Ginger oil can cause photosensitivity, so avoid using it if you're heading out into the sun.

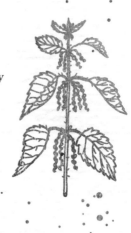

VETIVER (*VETIVERIA ZIZANIOIDES*)

If you run yourself ragged and need a little rejuvenation, vetiver can help. It calms an overactive mind, counters mental and physical exhaustion, and is used in Ayurvedic medicine for treating headaches. Its sweet and woody fragrance is said to dispel heat from both the body and the mind, likely one of the reasons for its calming effects and ability to temper irritability. Carry a bottle of vetiver with you, inhaling its essence when you need a bit of extra calm. And, as the fragrance of vetiver mixes nicely with a variety of scents, helping them last longer, experiment with blending it with your other favorite essential oils.

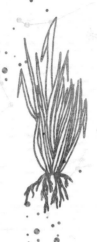

BLACK PEPPER (*PIPER NIGRUM*)

Pungent, *hot*, and *intense* are three words that can as readily describe an Aries as they can black pepper. This oil's warming properties increase circulation to the skin, help heal bruises, and relieve sore muscles. Its inspiring aroma can also lift your mood and energize your body. You can instill the atmosphere with some "rise-and-shine" energy by using black pepper oil in a diffuser. Or, add a drop or two to body lotion, and apply to sore muscles or bruised areas. Always dilute this strong essence in an oil or cream before applying it to your skin.

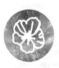 **Flower Essences**

Vibrational elixirs that catalyze psycho-emotional healing, flower essences are made from blossoms, perfect for Aries, since your sign represents budding growth. (See page 20 for how to use flower essences.)

IMPATIENS (*IMPATIENS GLANDULIFERA*)

Let's face it: as an Aries, patience isn't one of your strong suits. While you love the thrill of beginning new projects, you always itch to quickly move on to the next experience. When your creative undertakings don't wrap up in an expeditious manner, your patience can run thin, potentially leading to bursts of anger that may cause you, and those around you, undue stress. As its name implies, Impatiens flower essence is a perfect remedy to subdue the hot-tempered Aries' proclivity for impatience.

TIGER LILY (*LILIUM HUMBOLDTII*)

Known for being independent and pioneering, Aries are masters at expressing their will in the pursuit of a goal. Yet sometimes others may perceive your assertiveness as bordering on aggressiveness, which may dampen their desire to provide you with support and cooperation. Given the Ram's go-it-alone nature, this may not bother you as much as the next person. Yet there are still times when collaborative service is more efficient—let alone more enjoyable—than solitary action. If you want to transform a feeling that you're working *against* others into one in which you feel aligned to work *with* them, consider Tiger Lily flower essence.

LARKSPUR (*DELPHINIUM NUTTALLIANUM*)

The take-charge attitude and zest for life that Aries have make you born leaders, a role to which you are naturally inclined but that doesn't come without its own set of challenges. Sometimes the responsibility of being at the helm can weigh you down. Other times it is difficult not to slip into feeling an imbalanced sense of self-importance when given a position of authority. When you find it more stressful than joyful to motivate others toward a collective goal, consider using the flower essence Larkspur. It can help your natural leadership instincts bloom.

 # Yoga Poses

Yoga can provide another form of exercise through which Aries can channel their stockpile of energy. There are many different styles of yoga to practice, allowing you to indulge your desire for trying new things.

WIDE-LEGGED FORWARD BEND (*PRASARITA PADOTTANASANA*)

This pose allows you to experience having your head below your heart in a supported way. Thought to be good for headache relief, this pose brings blood to the head and calms the nervous system.

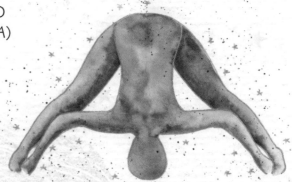

Standing tall with your hands on your hips, walk your feet 4 feet (122 cm) apart from each other, keeping them parallel. Gently hinge forward from your hips, keeping your back straight and placing your hands on the floor beneath your shoulders. Bend your elbows and allow your head to move toward the floor. If your head is close to the ground but can't reach it, place a folded blanket or yoga block underneath for support.

WARRIOR I (*VIRABHADRASANA I*)

Warrior I pose is perfect for the pioneering and champion-spirited Aries, reflecting the energy of the hero who conquers adversaries. This pose of strength and stability heats up the legs and moves the blood through the whole body.

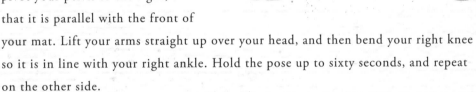

■ Standing tall with your hands on your hips, walk your feet apart so they are about 3 feet (91 cm) from each other. Turn your right foot to the right 90 degrees and your left foot 30 degrees in the same direction. Then pivot your pelvis to the right, so that it is parallel with the front of your mat. Lift your arms straight up over your head, and then bend your right knee so it is in line with your right ankle. Hold the pose up to sixty seconds, and repeat on the other side.

HEAD-TO-KNEE FORWARD BEND (*JANU SIRSASANA*)

This seated forward bend is calming to the brain and is said to relieve headaches and lower high blood pressure.

■ Sit on the floor on a folded blanket, with your legs straight in front of you. Bend your right knee and place the sole

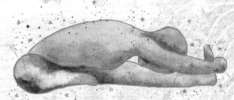

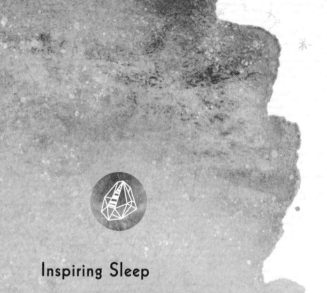

Inspiring Sleep

Aries are keen on short stints rather than lumbering through long hauls; therefore, one of the cardinal insomnia-battling strategies seems custom-made for you. After ten minutes of middle-of-the-night tossing and turning, get up out of bed, go to another room, and engage in a relaxing activity until the feeling of slumber returns; only then go back to your bedroom. What's powerful about this sleep-hygiene method is that it helps to disrupt any embedded association between your bed and sleeplessness that insomnia sufferers have.

of your foot against your inner left thigh, resting your outer right leg on the floor with your shin at about a 90-degree angle to your left leg (if your right leg doesn't reach the floor, place a folded blanket underneath to support it). Turn your torso to face your left leg. Grab your left foot with both hands (or use a strap if that is too challenging). Push your left thigh into the floor, extend through your left foot, and then bend forward to bring your extended torso toward your thigh. Hold for sixty seconds, and repeat on the other side.

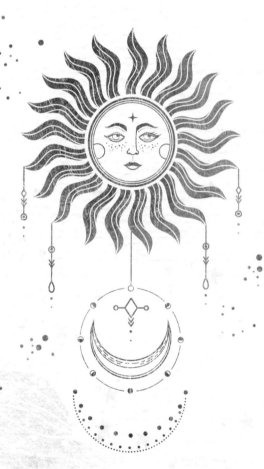

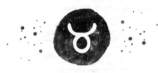

TAURUS

CHARACTERISTICS

Creative, grounded, kindhearted, patient, practical, predictable, security oriented, self-indulgent, sensual, serene, steadfast, stubborn.

SYMBOL

The Bull, an animal known for its strength, stamina, and grounded presence. Content on its own, it will become agitated if bothered by sudden movement. In mythological and cultural tradition, the Bull is a symbol of wealth, fertility, and stalwart power.

PLANETARY RULER

Venus, the brightest planet in the solar system. Venus was the Roman goddess of beauty and love, and represented sexuality, pleasure, and fertility. Her counterpart in Greek mythology was Aphrodite. In astrology, Venus represents love, beauty, and the force of attraction.

ELEMENT

Earth, which embodies the grounded energy of creativity, resistance, and practicality. It is fertile and passive, and it relates to the world on a sensual level. Pragmatism, routines, and sensuality energizes earth signs while fast movement, quick change, and an emphasis on sentimentality may deplete their vitality.

MODALITY

Fixed, which adores the planning and building phase of a creative project. Fixed signs prize reliability, predictability, and stamina. Discontinuity or too much change may throw them off their A-game.

Personal Health Profile

A Taurus has a hardy constitution and great physical resources. Like your astrological totem, the Bull, you are made of strong stock. Therefore, when it comes to keeping you well, your resilience is a strong asset. However, as a fixed earth sign, when you do get sick, it may take a while for you to fully recuperate, as Taurus needs time to rebuild their momentum and regain their grounding.

As stress greatly affects your physical health, keep in mind that change represents some of the most taxing conditions for the security-oriented Bull. When you feel that your sense of stability is being threatened or find yourself worrying about pending life changes, it's important to build in extra time to relax and pamper yourself.

Taurus is known for having highly attuned senses. Therefore, massages, body wraps, moisturizing treatments, and other sensually pleasing wellness therapies are sure to appeal to the tactile Bull, who likes to be pampered. Those born under your sign are more than willing to expend time and resources to take care of themselves, especially if the experience allows them to indulge their senses.

As the gourmets of the zodiac, Taurus loves food. Being so keenly aware of, and grounded in, your body, you're likely to be in tune with which foods will best meet your nutritional needs. However, your appreciation of food—and the pleasure it brings—may make it hard for you to stem your appetite. This may make maintaining an ideal weight a challenge for a Taurus, especially later in life.

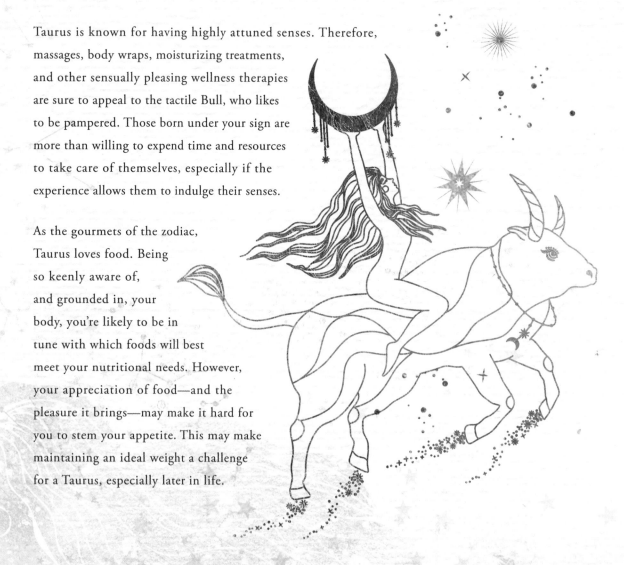

Not surprisingly, Bulls are famous for their bullheadedness, with a stubborn nature that makes it challenging to readily take advice from others, including health-care practitioners. Your routines are like a security blanket, and you hold on to them despite the toll they may take on your well-being. For your overall wellness, it's important to consider new health habits that may better serve your greater goals. And as much as change may be challenging, just think, once you get into the rhythm of these new ways, they'll bring you the comfort and peace of mind that comes from knowing you are doing the very best for your well-being.

 ## Areas of Health Focus

The parts of the body associated with Taurus include the following:

- The **throat**, which enables you to voice your truth

- The **neck** and **cervical spine**, which allow you to hold your head high

- The **inner ears**, through which you experience sound and a sense of equilibrium

- The **thyroid gland**, which regulates your metabolism

Your Taurean creativity, persistence, and practicality are some of the resources you can use when facing any health challenge.

PROTECT YOUR THROAT

The cold and flu season is a rather quiet time for Taurus; after all, it's difficult to make noise when you have a sore throat and laryngitis, common Taurean complaints. To maintain the health of the Taurus-ruled throat region throughout the year, adopt the habit of drinking plenty of water each day. Throat-soothing teas—many of which contain the herbs marshmallow root and slippery elm—with a touch of added honey make a delightful beverage. Also make sure your diet provides you with ample amounts of nutrients—notably immune-supportive vitamin C, zinc, and flavonoids—to help ward off infections.

PREVENT PAINS IN THE NECK

Taurus also governs the neck, making this part of your body a sensitive one, likely to play host to stress and tension. Luckily, you can do some practical things to help reduce neck stiffness and pain. Maintaining good posture—keeping your neck in a neutral position—is key. If you work at a computer, this means adjusting your desk and chair height so that the top of your monitor is at or just below eye level. Using a pillow with a shape that cradles your neck and supports its natural curve is also important. Doing gentle neck rolls and giving yourself frequent five-minute massages can help prevent neck cricks and discomfort.

GUARD EAR HEALTH

Taurus are all ears; you're a patient listener who sympathizes with others and their desire to communicate their values and needs. As your sign rules this part of the body, it's important to pay extra attention to your ears and protect your hearing. Ear infections or inflammation in this sensitive body part are often caused by allergies, sinusitis, or concomitant throat infections. Use earplugs when you're exposed to loud, potentially hearing-harmful sounds, whether from a concert or a neighbor's lawn mower. (Since a Taurus likes to always be prepared for the unexpected, keep a pack or two in your bag so they'll be handy when you need them.) For acute infections, try natural eardrops made from garlic, mullein, and St. John's wort.

SUPPORT THYROID HEALTH

Taurus rules the thyroid, the butterfly-shaped gland that produces hormones that regulate the body's metabolic rate. An overactive thyroid will result in your body burning energy too quickly while an underactive one can lead to a slowdown in metabolism, with ensuing weight gain. Thyroid imbalances often fly under the radar: they affect more than one in ten people, with women more likely to experience them than men. If thyroid hormone production is off kilter, it can affect your weight, mood, energy level, and menstruation cycle. If these symptoms ring a bell, it's worth discussing with your doctor, who can order a simple test to evaluate your thyroid hormone levels.

 # Healthy Eating Tips

As an earth sign, Taurus clearly understands how food can nurture their physical health while as sensualists you also derive much pleasure from food. As you're likely to be fixed in your ways, if you identify an eating habit you'd like to change, be patient and courageous in your undertaking.

LOVE FOOD WHILE LOVING YOUR HEALTH

When it comes to being the epicures of the zodiac, Taurus takes the cake. You love food—shopping for it, preparing it, and, of course, eating it. Food nourishes your senses, the Taurean GPS that helps you navigate your life. It also provides you with a feeling of being grounded, something that all earth signs crave. The obvious challenge for a Taurus food lover is preserving your culinary enjoyment while maintaining your waistline and health. To eat well and eat for wellness, shop at farmers' markets, where you can find heirloom and exotic varieties of fruits, vegetables, whole grains, and other nutrient-rich fare that will delight the gourmet in you.

ENJOY HOMEGROWN FOOD

Taurus, as an earth sign, is very connected to the land. Tending a garden and growing your own food, therefore, is something you probably dig. Plus, as a sign that appreciates the value of money, a Taurus will also treasure gardening as an economical approach to enjoying delicious vegetables, fruits, and herbs. Vegetable gardens let you experience the joy of nurturing the land and having it, in turn, nurture you through its bountiful harvest. If you are new to gardening, you can keep it simple by planting one or two types of easy-to-grow salad greens. Taurus apartment dwellers can exercise their green thumbs by growing windowsill gardens of culinary herbs.

INCREMENTALLY CHANGE YOUR EATING HABITS

A Taurus is a creature of habit. You derive great comfort from personal rituals, even if they are not the most supportive of your optimal well-being. For example, you may know that your afternoon triple latte isn't the best use of calories, but that doesn't make it any easier to forgo your three o'clock routine. A great way to override your hesitation to change is to dig your heels in and commit, knowing that in the end you'll be the better for it. Once you do so, use your stubborn and steadfast nature to your advantage to help you make the transition and stick to your new regimen. Pretty soon you'll get into the groove and the natural rhythms of your adopted healthful habit, comforted and supported by your new routine.

Health-Supporting Foods

Fruit and honey are both nutrient-rich ways to satisfy a Taurean sweet tooth. Very resourceful, the Bull may also appreciate using fresh garden herbs, since a little of each goes a long way to add flavor and health-promoting benefits to meals.

FRUIT

Eating a variety of fruit can help a Taurus bring their health goals to fruition. Fruit is a low-calorie way to curb sugar cravings, allowing you to stick to a diet while still indulging your desire for sweets. They are a source of quick, nutrient-rich energy that can put a spring in the step of the most grounded Bull. For optimal health, consume at least two to three servings of fruit each day. While juice can play a role in a healthy diet, don't treat it as a substitute for whole fruit, since it contains very little, if any, fiber and has less beta-carotene and flavonoid phytonutrients.

HONEY

Looking for an alternative to refined sugar? Consider honey. Not only does honey add sweetness to foods and beverages but it's also a whole food that contains antioxidant properties. In addition, honey mixed with warm water and a little lemon juice can offer much-needed relief from the sore throats a Taurus may experience. For greater nutritional benefits, including more antioxidant phytonutrients and cold-combating propolis, purchase raw honey rather than the pasteurized variety (unless you're pregnant or nursing, in which case raw honey is not recommended). Raw honey can be found in natural food stores and farmers' markets. Using local honey, produced closest to where you live, is thought to ameliorate allergy symptoms.

GARDEN HERBS

Parsley, sage, rosemary, and thyme: More than just a good lyrical refrain, this quartet of herbs can be one of the best additions to a Taurean menu. They're an inexpensive way to add flavor to your meals and, even when used in small amounts, they add a wealth of nutrients to your diet. In addition, they are easy to grow, something the practical and nature-loving Taurus will appreciate. You can garnish your health by including parsley in soups, stews, and salads. Add sage to your tomato sauce the next time you make pasta. Rosemary makes a great seasoning for chicken dishes. And, thyme is a flavorful addition to scrambled eggs and omelets.

 ## Wellness Therapies

Wellness therapies that delight your senses—especially those of smell, touch, and hearing—and that use natural, food-based ingredients are very healing for a Taurus.

AROMATHERAPY MASSAGE

An aromatherapy massage is perfect for the sensually oriented Taurus, as it indulges two of your senses—touch and smell—at one time. During this treatment, the practitioner prepares a custom-blended massage oil from fragrant aromatherapy essences that meet your specific wellness needs. For example, clary sage and rose oils are used to elevate energy levels, while lavender and chamomile oils are good for relaxation. If you have a penchant for certain fragrances, request them to be used in your treatment. You can benefit from this treatment at home by adding some essential oils to an unscented body oil and giving yourself a mini massage.

SOUND THERAPY

Taurus experiences the world through their senses, including hearing the sounds, and feeling the vibrations, all around them. Therefore, healing practices that incorporate sound may be perfectly tuned to your wellness needs. Techniques used by sound healers include special tuning forks, calibrated for different vibrations, that are applied to acupuncture points to bring about energetic harmony. Others may use Tibetan or crystal singing bowls that make use of the healing power of rhythmic sound waves. Another way to benefit from the healing power of sound is to participate in a sound bath, whether in person or online. Sound baths are like a meditation class in which the facilitator uses the ambient sounds to inspire very deep relaxation.

FOOD-BASED BODY TREATMENTS

As Taurus finds food so nurturing, why not let it also nourish your skin? Spas offer body-moisturizing regimens that feature natural ingredients such as coconut milk, avocado, and mangoes. Or enjoy an invigorating exfoliation treatment that uses pomegranate, rice bran, or cacao to help you shed dead skin. Not only do food-based body treatments offer a bevy of beauty benefits, but they also provide a calorie-free sensual feast. Remember, though, that when considering their services, it's important to let the practitioner know about any allergies you may have. For simple at-home treatments, use avocado for a facial mask, coconut oil as a body moisturizer, and very finely ground almonds to exfoliate your skin.

 # Relaxation Practices

Since Taurus needs to feel grounded and secure to be at ease, activities that connect you with the Earth can be very fruitful ways to relax.

POTTERY

Working with clay is a great way for the Bull to relax. It provides you with an opportunity to interact directly with an earth element, creating objects that have both beauty and function. Clay's malleability allows you to build and rebuild your pottery piece; from this art form, the fixed-nature Taurean can directly experience the power of change as a valuable part of creativity instead of a process to fear. The two main methods of creating pottery are wheel throwing and hand building. In wheel throwing, you sit at a potter's wheel and, aided by its spinning motion, shape the clay. Hand building offers a slower process that allows for greater control over the form you construct.

COMMUNING WITH NATURE

As an earth sign, Taurus enjoys being among the flora and fauna, which is key to developing a sense of inner peace. Whether you spend the day hiking in the hills or your lunch break strolling in a city park, getting out into nature will help you connect with the Earth's natural rhythms, which are ever so nourishing for you. In addition to walking, you can do many everyday things to keep connected to nature. Watch the birds take flight and listen to their magical songs. Plant your bare feet in the soil. Get grounded by digging in the dirt in your vegetable garden or flowerbed.

MUSIC

As a Taurus is acutely attuned to the aural realms, playing or listening to music can be an incredibly relaxing pastime. Music stimulates the throat and ears (in addition to the soul), parts of the body ruled by your sign. If you are caught in a labyrinth of looping thoughts, listening to music can help you find your way out. You can also try your hand at playing an instrument, whether you strum a guitar or beat on some bongos. Or sing, even if it's just when you're in the shower, to help you connect with your voice. Music is inspiring and experiencing sounds that you create is empowering.

Natural Remedies

Appreciative of the bounty that nature yields, Taurus understands the healing benefits that herbs, dietary supplements, and other natural remedies can provide.

MARSHMALLOW (*ALTHEA OFFICINALIS*)

If you get one of those pesky sore throats, try some marshmallow—the root from the *Althea officinalis* plant, not, unfortunately, the confection of the same name that lends its sweet gooeyness to campfire s'mores. Long used in traditional medicine to treat sore throats and coughs, marshmallow's botanical name is derived from the Greek word *altho*, which means "to cure." This throat-soothing herb is available in dried form or as a liquid tincture, either of which you can use to make a restorative tea. You can also find marshmallow as an ingredient in therapeutic tea blends that contain the herb slippery elm.

CHLOROPHYLL-CONTAINING SUPPLEMENTS

Chlorophyll allows plants to transform light into energy. It also gives plants their green color, reflective of the Earth and all its bounty. If your diet doesn't contain a lot of leafy green vegetables, you may want to consider adding a chlorophyll-rich food supplement—such as wheatgrass, barley grass, or blue-green algae—to your wellness repertoire. In addition to health-promoting chlorophyll, these supplements contain a range of other energy-producing nutrients. Green food supplements are available in liquid, tablet, or powder form, the latter being a great addition to smoothies.

HOMEOPATHIC BELLADONNA (*ATROPA BELLADONNA*)

Reflective of an association with Venus, your planetary ruler, *bella donna* means "beautiful woman" in Italian. Belladonna is a homeopathic remedy effective for many Taurean complaints, including sore throats, stiff necks, and earaches. It's particularly beneficial for those with stress caused by sudden movement, a characteristic of many Bulls. Homeopathic remedies are extremely diluted forms of the natural substance from which they are made; this is the reason that homeopathic belladonna is safe, but consuming the plant itself isn't. Mint and coffee can counteract the effectiveness of homeopathic remedies, so avoid them for several hours before and after taking belladonna.

 ## Essential Oils

Attuned to their senses, through which they navigate the world, Taurus can derive great pleasure from beautiful fragrances.

VANILLA (*VANILLA PLANIFOLIA*)

The essential oil of vanilla smells good enough to eat. Deliciously grounding and relaxing, vanilla is well known for its aphrodisiac properties, something that a sensual Taurus will appreciate. Mexican legend tells a tale of how vanilla came to be: a goddess, unable to wed the mortal she loved, transformed herself into a vanilla plant as a way to provide him with constant delight. Vanilla makes a lovely perfume either alone or mixed with other fragrances. Look for high-quality vanilla oil because the less expensive ones may be synthetically derived. If you can't find a pure essence, make your own by steeping chopped vanilla pods in jojoba oil.

PALMAROSA (*CYMBOPOGON MARTINI*)

Tall grass plants, like the one from which palmarosa essential oil is distilled, sway fluidly in the wind without losing their structural integrity. Palmarosa inspires this same feeling of secure movement in those who wear it, making it a perfect fragrance for the steadfast Bull. Endowed with a sweet citrus-rose scent, palmarosa is also used in many skin-care products for its antiseptic and moisture-balancing properties. When using palmarosa as a perfume, try dabbing some behind your Taurus-ruled ears. You can also put several drops in a mister bottle filled with water to make a refreshing skin toner, or add some to your moisturizer. When your feet get tired, soak them in a palmarosa-infused footbath.

THYME (*THYMUS VULGARIS*)

Throughout history, thyme has been heralded as an herb that promotes courage. Therefore, using thyme essential oil is good for a Taurus, whose slow-moving nature can sometimes use a little prod to push through barriers. Thyme can also be used as an antimicrobial agent, digestive aid, and scalp tonic. To benefit from its air-cleansing and mood-elevating properties, use thyme oil in a diffuser. Add a few drops to your shampoo bottle to enjoy its scalp-nourishing attributes. Thyme oil is very strong and may cause reactions if used directly on the skin; dilute it in oil, lotion, or liquid soap before using.

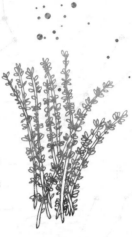

 # Flower Essences

Once you experience the healing results of flower essences and how they can help create balance on a psycho-emotional level, you will likely adopt these holistic remedies as a new wellness habit. (See page 20 for how to use flower essences.)

CHESTNUT BUD (*AESCULUS HIPPOCASTANUM*)

For a Taurus, the "been there, done that" idiom comes with a twist. For you, it's "been there, done that, now I'll do that again." More comfortable with the known than the unknown, you often repeat an action or stay with a habit even if it hasn't paid off in the past. The flower essence Chestnut Bud is perfect for times when you want a little help breaking free from a routine that provides you not with growth but only the comforts of familiarity.

IRIS (*IRIS DOUGLASIANA*)

Bulls have a keen creative flair. You have a visceral knowingness for what pleases the senses and the aptitude to create beauty from natural materials. Like many, though, you're probably intermittently plagued by doubt and what at times feels like an insurmountable barrier between yourself and your inner artistic spirit. When you're looking for the energy of a muse, try Iris flower essence. It can help reopen those channels of inspiration.

HOUND'S TONGUE (*CYNOGLOSSUM GRANDE*)

Taurus is a straight shooter who often lives by the adage: "What you see is what you get." As a practical and materially oriented sign, you take things at face value. Yet the complexities of life can sometimes call for going below the surface to examine the subtleties of a situation and the often hidden value that things inherently contain. When you need a little assistance delving deeper, going beyond a mundane-oriented understanding, try Hound's Tongue flower essence.

 # Yoga Poses

Yoga can be a great way for a Taurus to gain more flexibility. Poses that focus on the neck, cervical spine, and thyroid gland may be of particular interest to you.

COW (*BITILASANA*)

Named after kin of your astrological totem, Cow pose is perfect for the slow and steady rhythm of a Taurus. A great posture for coordinating movement with breathing, Cow pose enhances the flexibility of the neck and warms up the spine.

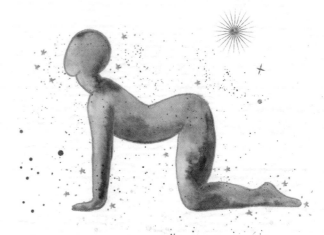

■ Place your hands and knees on
   the floor in tabletop position (your knees should align directly below your hips, with your elbows and wrists below your shoulders). Your neck should be in a neutral position with your eyes gazing toward the floor. While inhaling, lift your chest and sit bones toward the ceiling while dropping your belly to create a gentle arch in your back. Lift your head and look straight in front of you. Hold for several seconds. Exhale, draw your belly in, and move your spine back to tabletop position for several seconds. Repeat the sequence eight to twelve times.

BRIDGE (*SETU BANDHA SARVANGASANA*)

When your grounded nature needs an energizing lift,
try Bridge pose. This allover workout awakens the
senses and is especially beneficial for neck and
thyroid health.

- Lie flat on your back with your
  knees bent and your feet hip-width
  apart (or wider if your lower back is
  sensitive). To ensure proper foot placement,
  extend your arms along the ground, and place your heels in a spot that is several
  inches (centimeters) away from your fingertips. With your feet flat on the floor,
  slowly lift your hips. With your arms straight, clasp your hands behind your back.
  Stay in the pose for up to sixty seconds. When finished, gently roll down vertebra by
  vertebra on an exhalation.

STAFF (*DANDASANA*)

This pose, named for the straight rod-like positioning of your spine, is the foundation for
many other seated postures. While it seems basic, it has numerous benefits, including
energizing your whole body and stretching your neck muscles.

- Sit on the floor with your legs extended straight in front of you. Adjust your
  buttocks so your sit bones are on the floor (if your back isn't straight, consider
  sitting on a folded blanket). Without locking your knees, activate your legs by
  pushing your thighs into the floor and extending out through your
  flexed feet. Once your legs are engaged, press your hands into the
  floor to lengthen your spine so it is perpendicular to the floor.
  As you elongate your spine and find your inner lift from the
  tailbone to the crown of your head, widen your upper chest
  by rolling your arms away from your collarbones.
  Stay in the pose for at least one minute.

Inspiring Sleep

A Taurus is nurtured by reliability and routines. Whenever things seem stable and not apt to change, it leaves you feeling more grounded and secure. This aligns nicely with one of the key principles associated with getting better rest: maintaining a regular sleep-wake schedule and having the hours you get into bed and arise being somewhat uniform, even on weekends. Being able to honor your desire for consistency is key to keeping your body clock well regulated—and will be music to a Taurus' ears.

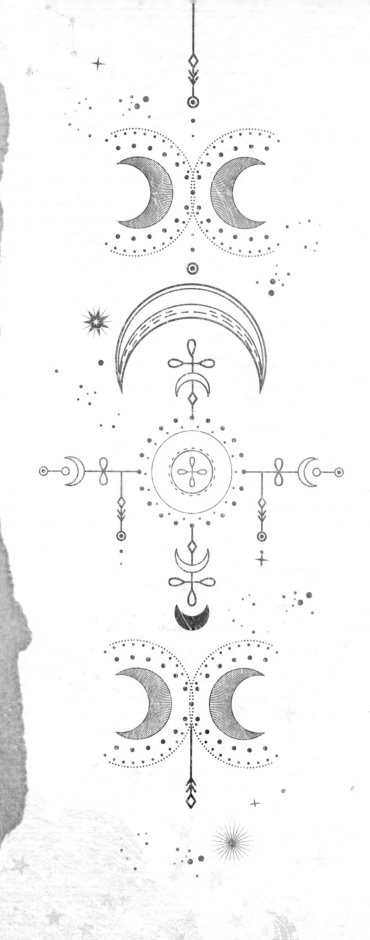

GEMINI

CHARACTERISTICS

Adaptable, cunning, curious, dual-natured, fickle, informative, mercurial, observant, quick-witted, spontaneous, talkative, youthful.

SYMBOL

The Twins, biological siblings who share a commonality while also expressing unique individuality. In mythological and cultural traditions, Twins are a symbol of the dualistic, yin and yang aspects that constitute the essence of the whole.

PLANETARY RULER

Mercury, which has the fastest orbit around the Sun. Mercury was known for his role as the messenger of the gods. His counterpart in Greek mythology was Hermes. In astrology, Mercury represents the mind, communication, and language.

ELEMENT

Air, which is associated with the agile energy of thoughts, observation, and logic. It is social, intellectual, changeable, and relationship oriented. Mental activities, communicating, and creating alliances energizes air signs while stasis, too much practicality, and heightened emotionality may deplete their vitality.

MODALITY

Mutable, which has an affinity for the adjustment and finessing stage of a creative project. Mutable signs are flexible, adaptive, and chameleon-like. They may find themselves agitated if things are too structured or overly defined.

Personal Health Profile

A Gemini loves to solve problems of all kinds, and those involving your health are no exception. With your keen curiosity and need-to-know nature, you'll wade through books, websites, and medical journals—and pick the brain of anyone in the know—in your quest to find the best treatment plan to cure your ailment or enhance your well-being. The road to wellness is an intellectual challenge that fascinates a Gemini. The process of finding the answer is as interesting to you as the answer itself.

While those born under the sign of the Twins like thinking about health solutions, committing to a plan composed of consistent actions can sometimes pose a challenge. One key to success is finding a wellness prescription that gives you a flexible structure while fulfilling your need for variety. For example, block off a specific window of time each day for exercising; then, depending on your mood, choose whether to walk, swim, practice yoga, or another of your favorite activities.

Also, when you try to solve a health conundrum, why limit yourself to one natural remedy or body-mind therapy? A well-researched assortment of self-care approaches will keep you from getting bored—the bane of a Gemini's experience—and will appeal to the various, and sometimes competing, aspects of your personality. (While the symbolic depiction of your astrological sign is a set of Twins, with the multitude of perspectives they hold, Geminis may sometimes feel more like octuplets.) One of the most beneficial yet challenging goals for a Gemini is to synthesize all parts of your multifaceted being. Therefore, an approach to health that honors your diversified preferences will not only prove interesting to you but healing as well.

Since Geminis are communicators par excellence, it's very important for you to find and work with health-care practitioners who match you on this level. Seek out those who listen well: not only are the Twins adept at describing their state of health in detail, but they also find the act of being listened to instrumental to feeling their very best. A great wellness guide for a Gemini is someone who provides you with plenty of information and resources. After all, knowledge is power—and the source of your personal empowerment.

 ## Areas of Health Focus

The parts of the body associated with Gemini include:

- The **lungs**, which provide your blood with the vital oxygen it needs to energize your body and mind

- The **nervous system**, the inner switchboard that processes information from your internal and external environments

- The **arms**, one of the twin parts of the body, from the shoulders all the way down to the fingers

Your Gemini communication skills, adaptable nature, and curious mind are some of the resources you can use when facing any health challenge.

SAFEGUARD RESPIRATORY HEALTH

As Gemini governs the lungs, you should take extra precautions to support respiratory health. Make sure to get an abundance of beta-carotene (a phytonutrient that the body converts to vitamin A) as well as vitamins C and E in your diet, as these antioxidant nutrients may protect against free radical activity in the lungs. If you have asthma or frequent respiratory colds, limit your intake of dairy products and food additives because these can exacerbate bronchial symptoms. If you want to curb congestion, try doing a steam inhalation using a few drops of eucalyptus, rosemary, or cedarwood essential oil. Also pay attention to your breathing—something a busy Gemini can forget to do—making it deep and rhythmic, because shallow breathing leads to reduced energy and a foggy mind.

RELIEVE STRESS AND TENSION

A Gemini loves to gather data; your restless, quicksilver mind seeks every possible fact and figure in your quest for knowledge. Yet, while you feel drawn to this type of mental stimulation, you can also suffer from information overload, resulting in undue stress on your nervous system. This strain may manifest in muscular tension—notably in the Gemini-ruled shoulders—as well as a state of low-level anxiety. To recharge your batteries and replenish your health, it's especially important for a Gemini to unplug every now and then; take periodic vacations from your cell phone, computer, and television, and schedule in a little quiet time each day when you can tune out the world and tune into yourself.

PROTECT YOUR ARMS

Geminis are masters of text messaging, remote controlling, mouse clicking, and gesticulating, all means by which you access and share information. What these activities also have in common is that they engage the arms in habitual motions that can tax muscles, tendons, and nerves, leading to repetitive stress injury. As you're unlikely to stop using electronic gadgets (or talking with your hands), safeguard your health by enhancing the ergonomics of your workspace. Invest in a mouse or trackball that cradles your hand, a functionally designed keyboard that allows for more natural wrist positioning, and a high-quality chair that features adjustable height and armrest positions.

WATCH OUT FOR ACCIDENTS

As a Gemini, you're likely very adept at multitasking. While performing many activities at once suits your restless and active spirit, it's not necessarily the best recipe for safety (especially if it's an activity that involves moving objects, such as talking on the phone while driving). Additionally, you may also run into problems—and three-dimensional objects—when you focus so intently on the inner landscape of your mind rather than the outer landscape of your environment. To mitigate an accident-prone nature, practice mindfulness, the art of being present in mind and body.

Healthy Eating Tips

For a Gemini, the trick to eating a healthful diet is to make it interesting, enjoying an array of different whole foods that offer your mind and senses a range of experiences.

EAT REGULARLY

Geminis dislike routine, and the idea of regularly scheduled meals may be no exception. When mealtime rolls around, you're likely to postpone it for something of more interest at the moment. The next thing you know, your blood sugar takes a nosedive and you grab anything, and everything, in sight with little regard to healthfulness. If you hate being pinned down to an exact mealtime, give yourself a more flexible two-hour window in which to enjoy your repast. If three squares a day doesn't work for you, consider five or six time-saving mini-meals. Regardless of the flexibility it features, having a somewhat consistent eating schedule is a good move when it comes to your physical health because it improves digestive function and better regulates appetite.

SLOW DOWN

When Geminis do get around to eating, they often rush through it, regarding it as an unwanted distraction from their work project, social engagement, or social-media scrolling. If you eat too fast, it can make your nerves jumpy, let alone lead to less-than-optimal absorption of nutrients. Eating slowly is not only a great mindfulness practice but can also help promote better nourishment. To make your meals more interesting, and help you more slowly savor them, combine foods that feature an assortment of colors, tastes, and textures. You can also put your Gemini scribe into action, using it to enhance your mealtime mindfulness; keeping a journal with you at meals and writing down your impressions of your culinary experiences is a great way to enhance your awareness.

STOCK THE BASICS

It's easy to identify a Gemini's kitchen. It's the one chock-full of condiments—a slew of salsas, an assortment of olive oils, a bounty of jams and jellies—and little else. Even if your cornucopia of condiments rivals that of the best gourmet stores, without some pantry basics, it's difficult to make a satisfying and nourishing meal. In addition to condiments, stock your kitchen with some nutrient-rich foundation foods to ensure that you always have the makings of a healthy and easy-to-prepare meal. Some of the basics include frozen vegetables, canned beans, brown rice, pasta, nuts, onions, and garlic.

 # Health-Supporting Foods

The Twins need variety in their diet so that they don't get bored of eating healthfully. Luckily, some of the best Gemini foods—orange-colored fruits and vegetables, oats, and dairy-free milk alternatives—can be prepared and enjoyed in a range of different ways.

ORANGE FRUITS AND VEGETABLES

Beta-cryptoxanthin, an up-and-coming nutritional star, is a cousin of beta-carotene that offers great support for the health of the Gemini-ruled lungs. It's a powerful antioxidant that can be converted in the body to vitamin A and is thought to lower the risk of developing lung cancer. And while beta-cryptoxanthin may be hard to pronounce, you can easily identify foods rich in this phytonutrient: just look for deeply orange-colored fruits and vegetables. Carrots, butternut squash, pumpkin, papaya, sweet potatoes, and tangerines are among your best bets if you would like to enjoy this carotenoid's benefits.

OATS

Enjoying a bowl of oats—served hot as oatmeal or cold as muesli—is a great way for a Gemini to start the day. Not only do oats have cholesterol-lowering benefits, but they are also thought to help soothe frayed nerves. Additionally, research suggests that a breakfast containing oats—a food governed by your planetary ruler, Mercury—can contribute to enhanced cognitive performance and sustained energy throughout the day. Instead of instant oatmeal, opt for rolled oats, which only take a few minutes to prepare but are much more nutritious. Add variety to your morning meal by alternating how you prepare the oats: try a sweet version topped with fruit and honey or a savory one mixed with spices and steamed vegetables.

DAIRY-FREE MILK ALTERNATIVES

While cow's milk and other dairy foods may be rich in calcium and other nutrients, many people are sensitive to them, leading to gastrointestinal upset and skin outbreaks. Plus, asthma and other complaints of the Gemini-ruled respiratory system are often linked to dairy allergies. If you're prone to these conditions, you may want to limit your intake of dairy products (or avoid them completely for a while) to see whether your health improves. If you're looking for dairy-free calcium contributors, try collard greens, kale, and spinach. You can find plenty of milk alternatives in the marketplace, including those made from almonds, hemp seeds, and, of course, oats. Some people with cow's milk allergies can tolerate goat's milk and products made from it.

 # Wellness Therapies

Many wellness therapies allow Geminis, so often in their minds, the ability to feel more grounded in their bodies, while others can help them probe the mines of their mind even further to gain valuable insights.

MANICURES

Geminis' hands are their ambassadors to the world. They help you write, collect information, and meet and greet the many people with whom you interact. Plus, as the zodiac's premier gesticulators, Geminis rely on their hands to help them communicate and express their thoughts. So, put your best hand forward by treating yourself to regular manicures. You don't have to spend too much money or time to keep your nails in tip-top shape; many salons offer express sessions that can give your hands a tune-up in a matter of minutes. Or you can do a manicure at home. A good place to start is by shaping your nails like a pro: file them from side to center in one fluid movement rather than using a back-and-forth motion. Keep a nail file in your bag so you can have it on hand for on-the-spot touch-ups.

CHAIR MASSAGE

A wellness therapy that requires a minimal time requirement, chair massage is tailor-made for a Gemini. It usually lasts only fifteen minutes, so you can enjoy one without taking too much time away from the many other things on your to-do list. During this treatment, you rest fully clothed in a padded chair that allows you to relax your upper body. In addition to massaging your neck and back, the practitioner will work out the kinks and stress residing in your Gemini-ruled shoulders and arms. Look for chair-massage kiosks in malls and airports. Or, serve up a DIY self-massage by lying on the floor with a tennis ball underneath your shoulder blades and rolling it around slowly to release pressure points.

TALK THERAPY

Gemini's planetary ruler, Mercury, is named after the winged-foot messenger god of Roman cosmology who readily crossed between the Earth and the underworld during his appointed rounds. Geminis are adept at this mercurial skill of traversing boundaries, which can be used to create a dialogue between the different levels of your mind. This gift, combined with your natural loquaciousness, makes talk therapy a natural choice for a Gemini. You can choose from numerous forms of talk therapy, including cognitive behavioral, psychodynamic, and others. Take time to do research so you can find the approach and practitioner that is the best fit for you.

 # Relaxation Practices

Reflecting the opposing yet complementary Twins that symbolize your sign, both stimulating and centering your mind can be relaxing to a Gemini.

GAMES AND PUZZLES

Participating in games and doing puzzles are great activities if you want to unwind. Plus, a night of games can be a fun activity for a social get-together, something the Twins cherish. And with the array of apps now available, it's also easy to virtually connect with others to play games and puzzles. One example is doing a jigsaw puzzle, which will not only exercise your spatial capacities, but also offers built-in flexibility, as you can finish the puzzle on your own timetable—a bonus for the busy Gemini. When you can't get friends or family together to play a group game, don't despair; working a crossword puzzle or playing an old-fashioned game of solitaire can be a very meditative experience.

PRANAYAMA

Pranayama is the Sanskrit name used to describe various breathing exercises practiced in the yogic tradition (*prana* means "breath" and *ayama* means "restraint"). Doing pranayama helps expand concentration while calming the mind and is often done before meditation.

It can also increase your awareness of your respiratory patterns, helping you catch any tendencies you may have toward shallow breathing. If you want to learn a few pranayama exercises, yoga classes are a great resource, as they usually include some breathwork practice. Plus, while you do *asanas* (poses), most yoga teachers will invariably remind you to concentrate on your breath. Yet, this practice is not limited to this tradition; there are a host of practitioners offering breathwork classes, both in person and online.

JOURNALING

Keeping a journal is a very helpful exercise for inventorying your thoughts and feelings. Whether it be stories, poems, or just random mind chatter, getting the words and ideas out of your head and onto the page—or the computer screen—can be a centering exercise for a Gemini. Your journal need not be limited to words; feel free to sketch or doodle too, if that helps you better express yourself. For a journaling practice that can help you more clearly access your subconscious, try nondominant handwriting: righties use their left hand, and lefties use their right. While your writing may look like kindergarten scrawl, you'll be amazed at how it can quiet your mind and draw out some under-the-surface memories.

57

 # Natural Remedies

Geminis may find it fascinating to learn about all the different natural remedies they can use to customize their self-care regimens.

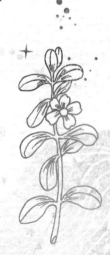

BACOPA (*BACOPA MONNIERI*)

A Gemini loves to discover new things, and if it's something like the herb bacopa, which helps enhance your memory and concentration, all the better. While recent research studies have discovered it to have promising neuroprotective and cognitive-enhancing effects, bacopa has benefits that are anything but new. This herb has been used for more than three thousand years in Ayurvedic medicine, where it is classified as a *medhya rasayana* (mind rejuvenator). You can find bacopa in pure herb form or standardized to levels of bacosides A and B, two of its active compounds. In addition to using it as a supplement, bacopa extract is mixed with massage oil and rubbed into the scalp as a stress-relieving treatment in Ayurvedic practice.

B-COMPLEX VITAMINS

B vitamins have a range of functions, including supporting energy production and maintaining the health of the nervous system. If your diet is not replete with whole grains, leafy greens, and legumes, you may want to consider taking a B-complex supplement, or at least be certain your multivitamin provides adequate amounts of these nutrients. Some medications—including oral contraceptives and estrogens—deplete the body's store of B vitamins, making it even more important to ensure you get enough. It's thought best to take B vitamins with food to avoid stomach upset. As with all supplements, let your doctor know if you're considering a B complex so you can discover any interactions it may have with medications you may currently take.

KALI MUR CELL SALT

Kali mur is the name of the homeopathic cell salt made from potassium chloride, a mineral found in muscle, nerve, and brain cells. Associated with Gemini, this cell salt is involved in the expression and dispersion of energy. When anxiety and nervousness manifest and cloud mental clarity, kali mur is often suggested as a good remedy. Cell salts like kali mur are available in health food stores and natural pharmacies. Mint and coffee can counteract the effectiveness of homeopathic remedies, so avoid them for several hours before and after taking kali mur.

 # Essential Oils

That the aromas of essential oils are not only pleasing but can also have profound effects on health may be an enchanting idea for the mind of a Gemini.

ROSEMARY (*ROSMARINUS OFFICINALIS*)

Since antiquity, when ancient Greek scholars wore rosemary wreaths to aid their studying, this herb has been esteemed for its ability to inspire concentration and fortify memory. Its rosmarinic acid component helps calm the nerves, making it a relaxing tonic for a Gemini. To benefit from a concentration-enhancing halo, mix a few drops of rosemary essential oil into your hair conditioner. Keep a bottle of rosemary on your desk, inhaling it any time you want to release stress and enhance your focus. Grow a rosemary plant on a sunny windowsill and enjoy its aroma in your tea or lemonade.

LAVENDER (*LAVANDULA ANGUSTIFOLIA*)

Like the Twins, Mercury-ruled lavender seems to have two different sides when it comes to its benefits, both of which reflect the very useful properties of this popular essential oil. Part of its attractive quality comes from its sweetly floral and relaxing scent, making it a favored perfume. The other facet of its attractive quality—to bugs, that is— makes it a powerful microbial agent and insect repellent. Lavender is a lovely scent to wear as a natural perfume; add some to your body lotion, or dab a few drops mix with jojoba oil on your neck or wrist. You can also fill a small cloth bag with dried lavender buds and use it as a drawer sachet to fragrance your clothes and keep pesky moths away from your prized sweaters.

EUCALYPTUS (*EUCALYPTUS GLOBULUS*)

Eucalyptus essential oil makes a great addition to a Gemini first-aid kit. It is well known for its respiratory health properties: not only is it an effective expectorant, but research suggests that it also has potent antimicrobial action against bacteria that cause bronchial infections. This fresh-smelling oil can also help ease muscle aches and pains. To relieve congested lungs and nasal passages, fill a basin with hot water and add a few drops of oil, and do a steam inhalation treatment. You can also mix some eucalyptus with coconut oil for an invigorating chest-rub ointment to help with respiratory ailments.

 # Flower Essences

If you want to learn more about ways to balance your emotions and transform psychological challenges into strengths, flower essences are a great thing to investigate. (See page 20 for how to use flower essences.)

WHITE CHESTNUT (*AESCULUS HIPPOCASTANUM*)

A Gemini's mind usually spins with ideas. While numerous thoughts circulate through for your analysis and reflection, sometimes a particular one may get stuck—repeating itself again and again—in what seems like a perpetual mental merry-go-round. If you need help calming mind chatter and breaking the reins of looping thoughts, try White Chestnut flower essence.

COSMOS (*COSMOS BIPINNATUS*)

Geminis are lifelong curators of facts and figures. While your mind's gallery contains a vast collection of information, synthesizing the pieces into a whole can be a challenging pursuit, even for the intellectually oriented Twins. Cosmos flower essence helps focus the mind and create a clear channel between thoughts and the spoken words used to express them. As such, it can be a great aid for public speaking.

CERATO (*CERATOSTIGMA WILLMOTTIANUM*)

A Gemini's love of information often translates into seeking insights from other people—usually lots of other people. Yet if you rely on the advice of others too frequently, especially as a substitute for trusting your inner voice, it can lead to confusion. Or worse, it can result in your acting in ways counter to your own true nature. When you need a little boost of confidence in your own decision-making abilities, Cerato flower essence may be a good option.

 ## Yoga Poses

The mindfulness-enhancing practice of yoga can help enhance a Gemini's innate sense of flexibility, giving you an opportunity to move your body and feel centered in it.

COBRA (*BHUJANGASANA*)

This mini backbend is a great pose for reversing the effects of the slouching shoulders and compressed chest that can arise after hours engaged in writing, surfing the Internet, catching up with friends online, or other activities that communicative Geminis favor.

- Lie face down on your mat, legs hip-width apart, with the tops of your feet touching the floor. Place your hands on the ground next to your chest while keeping your elbows close to your body. On an inhalation, ground your legs and press your feet down into the floor (where they should remain). Simultaneously, press through your palms, lifting your chest in a slightly backward arc. Roll your shoulders back and down, and lift through your sternum, which will help you avoid compressing your lower back. Stay in the pose for up to thirty seconds. When ready to leave the pose, exhale, and come down slowly.

EXTENDED SIDE ANGLE (*UTTHITA PARSVAKONASANA*)

Extended Side Angle pose stretches and strengthens many parts of your body, including the shoulders, arms, and wrists. It's challenging to perform, let alone master, which is an extra perk for puzzle-solving Geminis.

■ Standing tall with your arms outstretched to each side and your palms facing upward, walk your feet apart so that they are about 4 feet (122 cm) from each other. Rotate your right foot 90 degrees toward the right and your left foot 45 degrees in the same direction. Bend your right knee so that your calf is perpendicular to the floor and your knee is over your ankle. Tilt your torso and pelvis to the right, and place your right forearm on your right thigh. Stretch your left arm over your ear and toward the right side so that you feel a lengthening through your left torso while trying to keep your right torso lengthened as well. Stay in the pose for up to sixty seconds, and then repeat on the other side.

DOLPHIN (*ARDHA PINCHA MAYURASANA*)

Like a Gemini, dolphins are considered to be extremely intelligent. If you seek a posture that will help you stretch and strengthen your shoulders, arms, and wrists, Dolphin pose is a smart choice.

Inspiring Sleep

Your intense intellectual curiosity is one of your strengths; yet, if your Gemini mind is racing with thoughts and ideas when your head hits the pillow at night, it can be an obstacle that keeps you from getting a good night's sleep. Given that your sign rules the respiratory system, doing simple breathing exercises before slumber may help calm your mind and ease your transition to the land of Nod. White Chestnut flower essence (see page 60) may also help mollify any mental merry-go-round action that's keeping you from drifting off to sleep.

■ Place your hands and knees on the floor in tabletop position (your knees should align directly below your hips, with your elbows and wrists below your shoulders). Drop your elbows to the floor underneath your shoulders. Keeping your elbows in place, interlace your fingers together. Tuck your toes under, and send your hips toward the sky while pressing your forearms and wrists into the ground. The crown of your head should be facing the mat and contained within the triangle-shaped space created by your arms. Your knees can be straight or slightly bent, whichever allows your pelvis to lift away from your shoulders. Stay in the pose for up to sixty seconds.

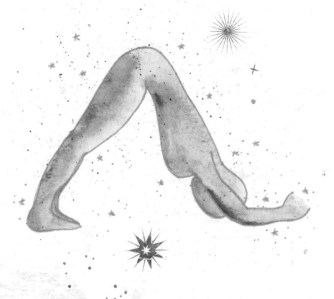

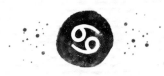

CANCER

CHARACTERISTICS

Defensive, emotional, gentle, hospitable, indirect, kind, moody, nostalgic, nurturing, protective, sensitive, traditional.

SYMBOL

The Crab, an animal known for both its hard shell that protects a soft interior and its claws that defend and gather food. In mythological and cultural traditions, the Crab is a symbol of service, loyalty, bravery, and a nondirect approach to confrontation.

PLANETARY RULER

The Moon, known for its cycles and for reflecting the Sun's light. Selene was the Greek goddess of the Moon while her Roman counterpart was known as Luna. In astrology, the Moon represents feelings, unconscious patterns, nurturance, and maternal instincts.

ELEMENT

Water, which embraces the fluid energy of emotion, reflection, and nonlinear understanding. It is sensitive, personal, and responsive. Feelings, empathy, and soulful connections energize water signs while excess rationality, lack of personal space, and inability to access their intuition may deplete their vitality.

MODALITY

Cardinal, which loves beginnings and the first stage of a creative project. Cardinal signs are motivated, ambitious, and enterprising. They encounter stress when things are not fresh and new.

Personal Health Profile

Despite a Crab's defensive shell, within you resides a very sensitive soul whose physical health is highly influenced by an expansive reservoir of feelings. On occasion, a Cancer may become captivated by a sense of moodiness that seems to come from nowhere, while in reality it springs from the deep sentimental undercurrents that live within. Accepting and expressing these emotions, rather than fearing and internalizing them, can do wonders for Cancerian health.

Cancers are very intuitive, often aware of—and able to remedy—symptoms of health imbalance before they transform into more serious concerns. You're also especially attuned to the cycles of the Moon, your planetary ruler. This lunar alignment makes Cancers cyclical creatures, whose moods, energy levels, and even water retention (and therefore, weight) wax and wane throughout the month. Knowing this about yourself is important in planning your health-care strategies. This wisdom can also provide calming to the Cancerian spirit by helping you realize that it is often periodicity, rather than unpredictability, that guides your feelings and physical health.

The Moon is the astrological symbol for the mother and, as such, represents feminine energy expressed through instinctive maternal sentiments. Cancers, in accordance with their planetary ruler, possess great nurturing qualities. Not only do you like to care for others, but you also like

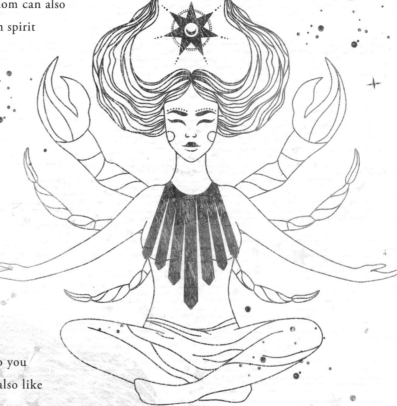

to be cared for; having another comfort you, even in the smallest of ways, can do wonders for your well-being. The trick to optimal health, though, is to refine your self-care abilities so you needn't be overly dependent on others.

With a strong reverence for all that came before you, Crabs are often very traditional creatures. Since your temperament is aligned with things that are tried and true, you're more likely to try one of the latest wellness trends if it's well rooted in the past. For example, folk remedies—including those handed down through the generations of your own family—appeal to your nostalgic orientation.

Your allegiance to time-honored traditions is bolstered by an inclination toward preventive medicine. The safety-seeking Crab is motivated to action by preservation and the reduction of perceived threats, illness included. Going to the doctor for routine visits is comforting to a Cancer, especially if your health-care practitioner is a nurturing and kind soul.

 ## Areas of Health Focus

The parts of the body associated with Cancer include:

- The body's containers, such as the **stomach** and **sinuses**

- The **esophagus**, the passageway through which food enters the stomach

- **Digestive juices**, **saliva**, and other **body fluids**

- The **breasts** and **womb**, symbols of femininity and nurturance

Your Cancerian caretaking nature, strong sense of intuition, and desire for self-protection are some of the resources you can use when facing any health challenge.

TRUST YOUR GUT

In medical astrology, the stomach and esophagus are ruled by Cancer, making them two of the spots to which the Crab may want to give a little extra TLC. Reducing caffeine, watching out for food allergies, and eating slowly can help reduce heartburn, as can the dietary supplement bromelain and the herb slippery elm. While excess stomach acid can cause challenges, so can insufficient amounts. Often an outcome of the routine use of antacids, low stomach acid (hypochlorhydria) can lead to indigestion as well as malabsorption of protein, vitamin B12, and other nutrients. Bitter herbs such as gentian may be helpful for stimulating gastric acid production. Additionally, a Cancer's stomach may often be tied in knots, especially if you tend to internalize your feelings rather than express them. Making time each day to relax can help pacify butterflies and calm a nervous stomach.

SOOTHE YOUR SINUSES

Sensitive to their environment, Cancers may be allergy sufferers. And with your sign ruling the sinuses, allergies—as well as infections—that affect this part of the body may be common fare. The traditional route to quelling sinus infections includes antibiotics and decongestants. A preventive approach includes supplements such as n-acetylcysteine and vitamin C. The Ayurvedic practice of *jala neti*, nasal irrigation using a neti pot, can also be helpful for relieving sinus congestion. Additionally, watch out for food allergies; while Cancers may gravitate toward milk and other dairy products because of their soothing texture, these foods provoke sinusitis in some people.

REDUCE WATER RETENTION

Not only do Crabs cling tightly to their feelings and possessions (and the past), but your body may also hold on to excess water. To curb a tendency toward swelling and bloating, avoid overly salty foods and drink adequate amounts of filtered water. As potassium helps with fluid balance, make sure you get adequate amounts of this mineral through your diet. Vegetables and fruits—especially leafy greens, melons, citrus fruit, and, of course, bananas—are among the best choices because they provide you with the greatest amount of potassium per calorie.

MAINTAIN BREAST HEALTH

Since Cancer is the sign of the mother, it's not surprising that breasts are under its domain. If you're prone to fibrocystic breast condition, dietary strategies can be of great benefit; eliminating (or at least reducing) caffeine and limiting saturated fat-rich foods like red meat can help with breast tenderness. In addition to regularly scheduled gynecological appointments, monthly self-exams are an important strategy for early breast cancer detection. If you have issues with your breasts—their size and/or shape—you're not alone. While many women wish their breasts were different, the first step in taking the best care of your breasts is to appreciate them—and the beauty of their uniqueness—as they are.

 ## Healthy Eating Tips

Cancers gravitate toward food; after all, yours is the sign of nourishment and nurturance. While food can provide you with comfort, be aware of becoming too reliant on it for soothing wistful moods.

BE AWARE OF EMOTIONAL EATING

Cancers equate the act of eating with the act of being nurtured. Food can feed the Cancerian soul, and eating is part of your self-soothing repertoire. But therein lies the rub: as sensitive Cancers frequently look for consolation, emotional eating can often lead to overeating. There is actually nothing inherently wrong with feeling nurtured by food—in fact, experiencing a sense of comfort from your meals is an integral facet of fostering well-being. It's just important to avoid using food as a panacea for your problems. If you find yourself eating to soothe anxiety or to satisfy an oral fixation, instead try chewing gum or snacking on carrots, celery, or other low-calorie, healthy finger food.

LOVINGLY PREPARE YOUR FOOD

The Crab loves to cook. For you, it's not just that home is where the heart is; the heart is where the hearth is. So, nurture your body while you nurture your spirit by cooking your own meals whenever you can. As you cook, focus on the food, infusing it with the abundant love you carry to further enhance the nourishing comfort it can provide you and others. Cooking your own meals doesn't mean having to spend a lot of time in the kitchen. There are many cookbooks available that can help you prepare quick, easy, and healthy meals in a matter of minutes. When you do go to restaurants—whether to dine in or take out—see if you can meet the chef, or at least peek in the kitchen to see who's cooking, as it can help you feel more connected to your food.

COOK WITH YOUR MELTING POT

As a Crab, your sense of security is closely tied to your family tree. The past, including who and what came before you, provides you with a strong sense of rootedness. Nurture the link to your lineage by taking a cooking class or buying cookbooks based on meals from your ethnic background or cultural heritage. In addition, consider compiling a collection of your family's favorite old-world recipes. Also, a trip to an ethnic food market can help you find ingredients as well as a piece of your cultural identity. Conversations with store owners may give you additional insights into traditional recipes and cooking methods.

 # Health-Supporting Foods

Included among the nourishing foods for the Crab are brassica vegetables and fermented soy foods. Often looking for foods with soothing textures, a Cancerian may appreciate Moon-ruled summer and winter squash.

BRASSICA VEGETABLES

Family is important to a Cancer, and the brassica family of vegetables—including broccoli, cabbage, cauliflower, watercress, and mustard greens—can be important to your health. Also known as crucifers, their unique sulfur-containing nutrients help the liver neutralize cancer-causing chemicals. This could help explain why research has suggested that women who regularly eat brassica vegetables have a lower risk of developing breast cancer. Steamed broccoli or cauliflower drizzled with extra virgin olive oil and a touch of lemon juice makes a quick-and-easy side dish. Watercress and mizuna (Japanese mustard greens) are great additions to salads. Sauerkraut and the Korean staple kimchi are delicious cabbage-based dishes.

FERMENTED SOY FOODS

While soy foods may not be the magic bullet that some claim them to be, they are versatile and tasty diet additions with health benefits that should not be discounted. Soy foods help promote bone health and lower cholesterol, and if consumed during adolescence, are thought to reduce breast cancer risk. To get the most from soy foods, enjoy them as they're consumed in Asia, where they're prepared with traditional fermentation processes and eaten in moderation. Eat whole soy foods—notably tempeh, miso, and natto—rather than soy-derived ingredients, like soy protein isolate and texturized vegetable protein. Look for products made with organic soybeans, which are GMO-free.

SQUASH

Squash is a Cancerian, Moon-ruled food that you can enjoy all year long. Summer squash, including zucchini, is low in calories and very filling. It's wonderful raw as crudités or sautéed as a delicious side dish. Winter squash features a comforting creamy texture and a sweetness that will help curb sugar cravings. Experiment with the many varieties of winter squash, including kabocha, sugar pumpkin, and delicata in addition to the old standbys of acorn and butternut. Steaming is a quick way to cook winter squash and cutting it into small cubes reduces the cooking time to less than ten minutes.

 ## Wellness Therapies

Wellness therapies can nurture your body and soothe your soul. Treatments that involve bathing provide a nourishing sense of aquatic cocooning precious to the Crab.

HYDROTHERAPY

Just like for your totem, the sea-dwelling Crab, water is the *prima materia* of your being. So why not soak up the many health benefits of this fundamental elixir by treating yourself to a hydrotherapy session? Also known as balneotherapy, hydrotherapy is a catchall phrase for healing treatments—such as underwater massages and mineral-rich soaking tubs—that involve water. There are many ways to benefit from hydrotherapy at home, such as making Epsom salt baths and foot soaks part of your regular wellness regimen. You can also alternate hot and cold running water in the shower for an enlivening and immune-system-boosting contrast hydrotherapy treatment.

MILK BATH

Take Cleopatra's lead and enjoy a luxurious skin-softening milk bath, a beauty ritual for which she was known. During this nurturing treatment, you soak in a tub filled with milk- and flower-infused water or have warmed milk poured over your body as you lie on a massage table (the benefits of this body treatment are thought to come from the milk's lactic acid, which gently exfoliates your skin). A milk bath is often followed by a body wrap, in which you're swaddled in herb-laden linens and left to rest. You can do a modified version of this treatment at home. Just add 1 cup (250 ml) of warmed milk and a few drops of your favorite floral essential oil—or a sachet of powdered milk and flower petals—to your bathwater.

JAVA LULUR

Java lulur is a spa treatment tailor-made for denizens of your sign; it is utterly feminine, incorporates the Cancer-ruled jasmine flower, and is steeped in tradition. This decadent therapy features a jasmine oil massage followed by a body scrub that includes jasmine, turmeric, and rice bran. After that, you're treated to a honey and yogurt body scrub and then a flower petal bath. While Java lulur is a time-honored ritual experienced by Indonesian brides-to-be, you needn't be prenuptial to enjoy its delights. Different spas have their own take on Java lulur, interpreting this ritual in a variety of ways; inquire about the spa's offerings (including time and cost) before booking a treatment session.

 # Relaxation Practices

Cancers can increase their state of peace by making time to nurture themselves, rather than just others, doing whatever it is that most pacifies their soul.

REGULARLY SCHEDULED "ME TIME"

Just like a Crab—which requires a quiet, undisturbed environment to molt and rejuvenate itself—you also need respites of peace and solitude to foster inner growth. It's important to carve out regular time away from attending to the needs of others so you can focus on yourself and do the things you love to do. Take a day (or even a few hours) off and laze in the bath, try out a new recipe, read a trashy novel, or do whatever floats your Cancerian boat. While many crabs molt every few months, you probably need to enjoy revitalizing "me days" a little more often. As Cancers are so in tune with lunar cycles, it makes sense to schedule your personal retreats at the New and/or Full Moon.

GENEALOGY PROJECTS

Your sign's deep connection to the past is an intricate part of your identity. To better understand your roots, why not dig up information on your ancestors and create a family tree? Talking to older relatives is a great place to start. Inquire about statistics—names, places, and dates—and also gather stories. For the nostalgic Cancer, the sentimental nature of genealogy can bring on a state of peace. A vast amount of genealogy resources are available on the Internet. In addition to numerous websites that will help you search through public records, there are discussion boards where you can get advice from others who are also researching their ancestry.

AQUATIC FITNESS CLASSES

For a Crab, exercising in your natural habitat of the water can be very relaxing. Aquatic fitness classes provide an opportunity for a cardiovascular workout that's safe, stress-free, and low impact—just the way a Cancer likes things. Moving against the resistance of the water, you build flexibility, endurance, and joint health. Aquatic fitness classes are designed for an array of energy and ability levels, so you will surely find one that best suits your needs. If you're not an avid swimmer, don't worry—in most aquatic classes, you usually wear floatation belts. If classes aren't available near you, you can always practice some aquatic exercises in the pool on your own.

 # Natural Remedies

As the sign associated with the mother, it makes sense that, to a Cancer, Mother Nature can yield healing treasures.

VITEX (*VITEX AGNUS-CASTUS*)

The Moon reflects the archetype of cycles, which are so intimately tied to femininity. Therefore, it's no wonder that your planetary ruler, the Moon, rules vitex, one of the premier herbs for women's health. It's used to promote well-being through numerous cycles of life, including for premenstrual syndrome, menstrual cycle irregularities, and menopausal symptoms. While vitex helps regulate hormone balance, it is actually hormone free. It's also known as chasteberry, reflecting the traditional belief that it inspired chastity by reducing sexual drive (don't worry, there's been no research to support such a claim).

BROMELAIN

As bromelain helps break down protein, these supplements are used as digestive aids. Bromelain has also been found to relieve symptoms of acute sinusitis. Since it also addresses many other ailments—including joint inflammation—bromelain is a great remedy to keep in your medicine cabinet. If you use bromelain supplements as a digestive aid, take it with meals; for other uses, it is best to take it on an empty stomach. As a way to ensure potency, look for bromelain supplements that report dosage in GDUs (units of activity) rather than just milligrams.

DEGLYCYRRHIZINATED LICORICE (*GLYCYRRHIZA GLABRA*)

Deglycyrrhizinated licorice (DGL) is a dietary supplement made from licorice. Its "de" prefix reflects that it is free of glycyrrhizin, a natural licorice component that can cause water retention and increase blood pressure. DGL can benefit a Crab in need of some stomach soothing, as it may help curb indigestion and heartburn. Research suggests that it may heal aphthous ulcers, a fancy name for the not-so-fancy canker sore. As DGL needs to be in contact with saliva to work, this supplement comes in chewable wafer form. Some companies sell DGL wafers that are flavored, a boon for those who don't like the taste of licorice.

 ## Essential Oils

That the oil derived from a flower, fruit, or herb is able to not only promote physical well-being but also elicit positive sentiments—from the joyful to the tranquil—is sure to please a sensitive Cancer.

JASMINE (*JASMINUM OFFICINALE*)

Jasmine is a flower governed by your planetary ruler, the Moon. Given that its sweet and intoxicating fragrance grows stronger as night falls and the Moon rises, its lunar relationship is not surprising. A powerful aphrodisiac, jasmine can help you open more deeply to your Cancerian-nurturing instincts while its rapturous scent can help lift your mood. You can enjoy the seductive fragrance of jasmine by wearing it as a natural perfume, or use jasmine-scented oil for a sensual couple's massage. If straight jasmine essential oil is not in your budget, a more affordable variety, diluted with jojoba oil, may also bring you joy.

HYSSOP (*HYSSOP DECUMBENS*)

Hyssop essential oil can help if your digestion needs a little jump-start or if you retain water during your period (or other times of the month). It's known as an "herb of protection," thought to help fortify the boundaries of those—like the Crab—who absorb other people's worries and stress. And for tradition-loving Cancers, it's nice to know that hyssop has been around for a long time, reflected by its mention in the Bible as an herb associated with purification. Use hyssop in a room diffuser to cleanse the air, especially if someone in your house is sick. Hyssop mixed with massage oil makes a great belly balm for upset stomachs or water retention. While several types of hyssop are available, many practitioners view the decumbens variety as superior.

CLARY SAGE (*SALVIA SCLAREA*)

Clary sage is a classical essential oil for women, used to relieve menstrual cramps as well as menopausal symptoms such as hot flashes. It is well known for its sweet and euphoric fragrance, which elevates moods and centers emotions. As its name suggests, it provides you with the wisdom of clarity, both in thoughts and in feelings. Clary sage is a wonderful essential oil to use during your period. Add some to your body lotion, and rub it onto your belly to alleviate the cramps and bloating that can accompany menstruation. A warm bath with a few drops of clary sage creates an enchanting relaxation ritual.

 ## Flower Essences

Flower essences, subtle remedies that work to balance emotional well-being, can help Cancers connect to their deep well of feelings, the source of their vital strength. (See page 20 for how to use flower essences.)

BABY BLUE EYES (*NEMOPHILA MENZIESII*)

Like your astrological symbol, the Crab, you likely have a hard, protective shell. Your defensive veneer helps you, an uber-sensitive soul, feel safe when you venture into the world. Yet this armor can sometimes keep you away from what you most crave: emotional connections with others. Baby Blue Eyes flower essence can help enhance your belief in your amazing intuitive nature, allowing you to let down your guard while still feeling protected.

CLEMATIS (*CLEMATIS VITALBA*)

As a daydreamy Cancer, you may sometimes appear to be "here"—present to the world around you—while you're actually "there"—burrowed in the feelings that reside within. While this withdrawal into the shell of your vivid internal life may appeal to your sensitive nature, it can sometimes keep you from facing tasks and achieving goals. When you need to bolster your ability to stay present within yourself and yet actively interact with the world, try Clematis flower essence.

HONEYSUCKLE (*LONICERA CAPRIFOLIUM*)

Cancers are nostalgic. The reliability of what came before gives you security, and the sense of being connected to your personal roots gives you comfort. While it's important to honor the past, a Crab may also have a tendency to get stuck in it, which can pull you away from truly living in the present. If you need a little help removing the pincer grip of the past, try Honeysuckle flower essence.

 # Yoga Poses

Yoga can be a gentle form of exercise that offers benefits for Cancer-related body parts such as the sinuses and stomach. As done in certain traditions, consider not practicing yoga on the New and Full Moons.

STANDING FORWARD BEND (*UTTANASANA*)

In addition to stretching the hips, hamstrings, and calves, Standing Forward Bend is good for enhancing the health of the Cancer-ruled sinuses and stomach. It's often referred to as Waterfall pose, well suited for your aqueous nature.

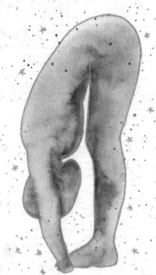

- Stand tall with your feet together or hip-width apart, whichever feels better. Place your hands on your hips. Bend forward from your hips, rather than from your waist. Bring your fingertips or palms to the floor in front of you, or rest your hands on your shins or block props. Regardless of your arm position, let your head hang down. Keep your legs straight without locking your knees (bend your knees if you have any discomfort in your back). Remain in the pose for up to one minute. To rise, either roll up through your spine one vertebra at a time or keep your spine long and come up in one breath.

EASY, WITH ALTERNATE NOSTRIL BREATHING (*SUKHASANA/NADI SHODHANA*)

This calming seated posture, wonderful in and of itself, is one that you can also use for meditation. Alternate nostril breathing is deeply relaxing and helps center the emotions.

- Sit on the edge of a folded blanket or yoga bolster that is 4 to 6 inches (4 to 15 cm) high to bring your pelvis into the same neutral position as if you were standing. Crossing your shins, open your knees to the side with your feet underneath opposite knees, and let your outer legs fall toward the floor. Press your right thumb on your right nostril to close it. Inhale through your left nostril for up to four counts. Close your left nostril with your right ring finger, release your thumb, and exhale through your right nostril for up to four counts. Inhale through your right nostril for up to four counts, and then close it with your thumb. Simultaneously release the hold on your left nostril and exhale for up to four counts. Continue for twelve rounds or more.

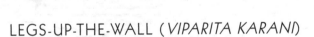

LEGS-UP-THE-WALL (*VIPARITA KARANI*)

This gentle, restorative pose inspires calm and relaxation, is thought to help with water retention, and can move blood through the stomach and reproductive organs. This allows you to gain the many benefits offered by other inversion postures without the intensity and stress they may cause.

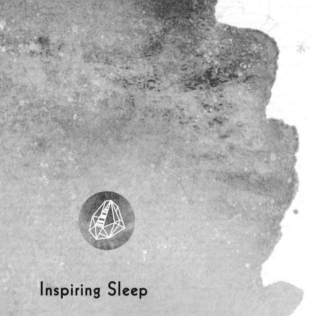

Inspiring Sleep

Home is so important to a Cancer. If it feels cozy and peaceful, it helps you to be more at ease and at home within yourself. To create more tranquility and help ensure you get a good night's sleep, you should treat your bedroom like a sanctuary, a place in which you feel safe and protected. To do so, make sure the décor feels nurturing, that you surround yourself with things that you love and cherish, and that the space is clutter free.

■ Sit on the floor with the right side of your body next to a wall and your legs bent and feet on the floor. Lie down so you are in a modified fetal position. Pivot yourself so you are lying on the ground. Straighten your legs and rest them on the wall, scooting your buttocks forward so that you are as close to the wall as possible. Rest your arms out to the sides. Close your eyes and relax for at least five minutes. If you need extra support, place a bolster under your lower back.

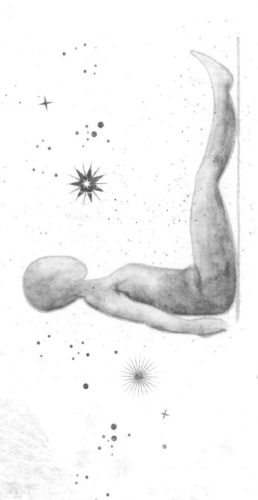

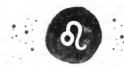

LEO

CHARACTERISTICS

Charismatic, cheerful, courageous, dignified, dramatic, expressive, faithful, forthright, magnanimous, proud, warmhearted, winsome.

SYMBOL

The Lion, an animal known for its lustrous mane and magnificent roar. As king of the jungle, the Lion is territorial, fierce, and powerful. In mythological and cultural traditions, the Lion is a symbol of strength, bravery, and royalty.

PLANETARY RULER

The Sun, a star at the center of our solar system that radiates heat and around which all planets orbit. The god of the Sun in both Greek and Roman mythology was Apollo, who governed truth, prophecy, and healing.

In astrology, the Sun represents the creative life force and a person's vital essence.

ELEMENT

Fire, characterized by the dynamic energy of inspiration, enthusiasm, and passion. It is transformative, kinetic, and action oriented. Movement, spontaneity, and tapping into their imagination energizes fire signs while slowness, stagnancy, and a sense of limitation may deplete their vitality.

MODALITY

Fixed, which adores the planning and building phase of a creative project. Fixed signs prize reliability, predictability, and stamina. Discontinuity or too much change may throw them off their A-game.

Personal Health Profile

Leos radiate an incandescent sense of wellness and vivacity. Roaring with stamina, you energetically participate in the many experiences life presents to you, including those that allow you to share your creative and shining self with the world.

With an ambitious and generous spirit, you may become overly fired up about the projects you undertake; this may be inspiring, and yet it can also sometimes be stressful, let alone exhausting. Luckily, your fiery nature and ability to find creative solutions will usually help you quickly rebound to your full-spirited energy level.

While Leos have an active and enthusiastic nature, it's important to recognize that you can sometimes fall prey to streaks of laziness. Let yourself enjoy these respites, although be aware if they cause you to stray too far from your dedication to exercise, eating well, and other aspects of your wellness routine.

The motivation of Leos to continually better themselves, in addition to their desire to take control of their own destinies, makes a self-care program of wellness therapies and natural remedies very attractive. Self-care lets you rely on your strong sense of agency rather than having to depend on others, thus allowing you to maintain the dignity so important to the proud Leonine soul.

Another reason Leos so willingly engage in self-care is that wellness therapies are enjoyable, especially the ones that involve pampering. What Leo doesn't love a day at the spa? You get to enhance your health and enjoy the treasures of sybaritic pleasure, all the while having someone lavish you with special attention. Being queen or king for a day (or even a few hours) is something to which regal Leos are drawn.

While Leos like to be in charge, when you do fall ill, it's important not to let your pride get in the way of asking for help. For a Leo, the ideal health-care practitioner is someone who will treat you as an individual—not just another patient—and who will respect you and your opinion. For a confident and engaged Leo, their shining their full attention on you (without being patronizing) can help you feel secure and best taken care of.

 ## Areas of Health Focus

The parts of the body associated with Leo include:

- The **heart**, which keeps blood flowing and symbolizes love and joy

- The **spine**, through which vital life-force energy moves

- The **hair**, an expression of your luster

Your Leonine creativity, courage, and ability to express yourself are some of the resources you can use when facing any health challenge.

CARE FOR YOUR HEART

Since the sign of Leo rules the heart, Lions may want to pay particular attention to their cardiovascular health. High blood pressure and atherosclerosis can cause your heart to work harder than it needs to. Your self-motivation is a plus here, as an individually guided wellness program of exercise, diet, and stress management practices can do wonders for heart health. Also important is being true to your Leonine nature: the Lion has a vast reservoir of love and affection, and by expressing your warm and generous nature, you can help keep your heart in regal condition.

SUPPORT YOUR BACK

The spine not only holds you up and gives you shape but it is also thought to be the channel through which vital life force energy flows. With Leo ruling the spine, the potential for back issues may be front and center in a Lion's life. As Leo is a fixed sign, maintaining flexibility—in both body and mind—is important and beneficial for those born under this sign. Look to yoga or similar forms of exercise to keep your back muscles supple (and your heart peaceful). If you have chronic back pains, movement-patterning approaches—such as the Alexander Technique or Feldenkrais Method (see page 154)—may be very beneficial.

GET SOME SUN

Sunshine is vital for a Leo's health. Your body is like one large solar cell, needing the rays of the Sun to charge your internal energy generator. So when the Sun doesn't shine—say, during the winter or in cloudy environs—you may find yourself prone to seasonal affective disorder, appropriately called SAD. These wintertime blues are characterized by low energy, mood lulls, and carbohydrate cravings. If spending winter in a tropical locale just isn't an option, don't despair. Full-spectrum lighting, regular exercise, vitamin D supplementation, and just getting out into the fresh air can do wonders for your emotional and physical health.

MAINTAIN YOUR GLORIOUS MANE

Lions are known for their manes, their noble crowns of hair, which communicate their prowess and stature. Similarly, as a Leo, your hair is likely to be one of the features you shower with a lot of attention and take great care in maintaining. While hair and scalp health require a range of nutrients, three key ones are protein, omega-3 fatty acids, and the B vitamin biotin. For a lustrous mane, regularly massage your scalp and deep condition your locks. And, as another reason to avoid stress, know that it can negatively impact your hair, as can certain medications and excessive alcohol intake.

 # Healthy Eating Tips

Leos enjoy life, and food and drink can definitely add to your pleasure; the challenge, of course, is not going overboard with overindulgences that can compromise your waistline and well-being.

EAT HEART-HEALTHY FOODS

To keep your arteries in top-notch shape, limit foods high in saturated fats—such as red meat—and shy away from synthetic trans-fatty acids found in hydrogenated oils. Some beneficial foods for heart health include omega-3-rich fish as well as nuts and seeds bursting with vitamin E. And, of course, enjoy an array of colorful fiber-rich fruits and vegetables, essential for cardiovascular health. For a meal to be heart healthy, avoid having saturated-fat-rich meat play the leading role; instead, when you do opt for it, let small portions (4 to 6 ounces [113 to 170 g]) costar on your plate with vegetables and whole grains. Create salads with a range of colored vegetables to enjoy a palette of different health-promoting phytonutrients.

BALANCE OUT YOUR FIERY ENERGY

As the sign associated with the Sun, Leos are hot, in more ways than one. In Ayurvedic medicine, an ancient system of healthcare that originated in India, a fiery constitution is known as *pitta*. When pitta becomes excessive, it can manifest in skin rashes, stomach acidity, inflammation, excess body heat, and irritability. If you find yourself overheating and faced with a short fuse, consider a cooling diet to balance excess pitta. Grapes and melons are very cooling, as are zucchini, cucumbers, broccoli, sprouts, and mint. While it may seem counterintuitive, avoid iced drinks if you have a fiery constitution; according to Ayurvedic medicine, too much cold can extinguish beneficial digestive fire, which can lead to indigestion and nutrient malabsorption.

CELEBRATE IN MODERATION

Leos love parties; after all, they're an opportunity for fun, one of your favorite pastimes. Yet parties—with their abundance of cocktails and canapes—can be challenging to your diet. It's easy to be so involved in meeting and greeting that you don't realize how much you're eating. At a gathering, enjoying a few nonalcoholic drinks will save you calories and won't dampen your fire the next morning. If sparkling water seems too dull, try a festive mocktail instead. Another pro tip: a light pre-party snack can curb your appetite and help you make non-impulsive food choices.

Health-Supporting Foods

Many delicious foods can help support the health of the Leo-ruled heart. Not surprising, some of these—including grapes and sunflower seeds—happen to be governed by your planetary ruler, the Sun.

GRAPES

Like a Leo, grapes need plenty of sunshine to flourish. Among their numerous benefits, grapes are a sweet way to keep your heart in tip-top shape. While green grapes are delicious, red and purple ones contain more antioxidants, including resveratrol (which is even more concentrated in red wine). This nutrient extraordinaire is a hot topic in research circles for its cardiovascular and antiaging benefits. Some people who are sensitive to red wine find that drinking natural wine (which is grown organically and avoids artificial additives during the fermentation process) doesn't cause them to experience headaches and other negative effects. If you want to steer clear of alcohol, enjoy grape juice or dealcoholized wine instead.

SUNFLOWER SEEDS

Not surprisingly, the sunflower—with its halo of brilliant yellow petals—is ruled by the Sun. The seeds of this majestic flower are one of the most concentrated food sources of vitamin E, which, by protecting LDL cholesterol (often referred to as the "bad" cholesterol) from oxidation, may help reduce the development of atherosclerosis. Sunflower seeds are also rich in phytosterols, plant-based nutrients that can lower cholesterol levels. Enjoy them as an addition to salads, cereals, and stir-fries. Or, try a heart-healthy SB&J sandwich made from sunflower seed butter and orange marmalade. While they may make a good snack, moderation is key because sunflower seeds contain about 400 calories per ½ cup (66 g).

OMEGA-3-RICH FOODS

A Leo's fiery constitution may create heat that exacerbates conditions of inflammation. Some of the best anti-inflammatory nutrients around are omega-3 fatty acids, which can support the health of your heart and hair, and help your skin defend against sunburn.

Among the richest sources of omega-3 fatty acids are salmon, flaxseed, chia seeds, walnuts, winter squash, and the wild green purslane. To enjoy more of this nutrient, top a salad of purslane and your other favorite greens with canned salmon; sprinkle chopped walnuts on baked winter squash; and add ground flaxseeds or chia seeds to cold cereal, oatmeal, or yogurt.

Wellness Therapies

Wellness therapies, especially those that leave you feeling pampered and well attended to, can be a very enjoyable part of a Leo's health-care regimen.

HOT STONE MASSAGE

Combine your fondness for being pampered with your love of heat, and enjoy a luxurious hot stone massage. By using smooth river stones that have been heated to a comfortably hot temperature, the practitioner provides you with a muscle-relaxing massage. The stones are also left to rest on different areas of your body—including along your spine, a special treat for Leos with back concerns. The stones' warmth melts away stress and tension, allowing the massage therapist to work deeper muscles without applying a lot of pressure. You can try a modified version of this treatment at home: purchase specially polished massage stones, heat them to a comfortable temperature in a pot of water, and apply them to different areas of your body.

BIOFEEDBACK

As a Leo, you have a great talent for gleaning insights from the world around you and using them for your own personal growth. That's what makes biofeedback such a great therapy for you. In a biofeedback session, body functions—such as heart rate or muscle tension—are measured and relayed back to you; you then focus on your intended goal—for example, relaxing your body—as you continue to receive feedback regarding your progress. Biofeedback is commonly used for alleviating hypo- or hypertension, chronic back pain, and tension headaches. There are an array of biofeedback devices that you can use at home, including wearable devices that measure your heart rate variability, and help you monitor your sleep and stress levels.

HAIR AND SCALP TREATMENTS

As Leos hold their manes in high regard, taking good care of your hair will help you feel your best. Many spas offer treatments, which you can enjoy alone or as an add-on to other services, specifically designed to encourage the health and beauty of your hair and scalp. Consider a deeply moisturizing jojoba oil treatment or a nourishing mudpack. If your hair has been damaged from too much sun exposure, try a Hawaiian-inspired treatment of coconut and kukui nut oils. If you don't have the time or money to make it to a spa or salon, pamper your hair and scalp at home with hot oil and deep-conditioning treatments. And don't forget about regular trims; it's the easiest way to take care of split ends and add sheen and luster to your locks.

 # Relaxation Practices

Leos are most at ease when they are able to shine brightly, expressing the warmth of their hearts and sharing their dynamic selves with the world.

SUNBATHING

For Leos, relaxing is simple: a beach chair, a book, and the Sun's warming rays are the perfect recipe for melting away stress. While ultraviolet rays will recharge your spirit, it's still important to practice good sunbathing habits. Invest in sunglasses with UV protection, and don't forget to wear a lotion with a minimum of SPF 30; after all, sunburns are anything but relaxing. If you can't get out into the sunshine, bring it—or at least a close approximation of it—to you. Consider getting a light box or brightening up your home and office by using full-spectrum light bulbs, which come in an array of styles that fit most types of lighting fixtures.

CHILD'S PLAY

Your playful Leonine spirit makes you a natural with kids. Spending time with children will remind you of how fun and uncomplicated life can be. It also helps you reconnect with your inner child and the zest that comes from seeing things with fresh, unadulterated eyes, allowing your heart to shine even more brightly. If you don't have kids of your own—or even if you do—consider volunteering with a children's organization. For example, many schools and nonprofits have programs through which you can tutor children or coach them in intramural sports.

ACTING

For you, Leo, the world is your stage, and every life event is an opportunity to be true to your passionately expressive nature. So why not tap further into your inner thespian—or drama queen—and take acting classes. Not only will you learn skills that will help you dig deeper into your essential creativity, but you'll have a lot of fun to boot. Acting classes offer a structured venue for being in the spotlight, enabling you to feel safe and supported, something Leos need to shine their brightest. As acting teachers have different styles, methods of teaching, and of course, personalities, see if you can visit several different classes before committing to one.

 # Natural Remedies

Leos like to be in charge, and using natural remedies provide you with another way to manage your well-being routine.

VITAMIN D

Vitamin D is known as the "sunshine vitamin" because the Sun's ultraviolet rays make it active in our bodies. Anything that causes reduced sun exposure—such as staying indoors, living in a cloudy climate, or wearing protective clothing—can put people at risk for vitamin D deficiency. Vitamin D is a hot topic in nutrition: while it was once famous solely for its contribution to bone density, this nutrient is now thought to also play a role in promoting heart health and ameliorating depression. To determine the optimal amount to supplement, ask your doctor about tests that can measure your vitamin D levels.

ST. JOHN'S WORT (*HYPERICUM PERFORATUM*)

St. John's wort is a remedy traditionally associated with Leo and your planetary ruler, the Sun. Most famously known for treating mild depression, St. John's wort may also benefit those who experience seasonal affective disorder (SAD), the blues that occur from a lack of sun exposure. A salve made from this healing herb can be used topically for calming sunburns as well as relieving bruises and skin irritations. St. John's wort is available in capsule, liquid tincture, or topical form. In some individuals, taking St. John's wort may cause photosensitivity (heightened sensitivity to the Sun), resulting in itching and redness.

CHAMOMILE (*MATRICARIA RECUTITA*)

Considering that its bright yellow flower head is surrounded by a corona of petals, it's not surprising that chamomile is traditionally associated with the Sun. Owing to its muscle-relaxant and antispasmodic properties, one of its traditional uses has been as a stomach soother. And when you feel overly agitated, either during the day or before sleep, you'll appreciate the calm it can impart. Applied topically in the form of a cream or an ointment, it may speed the healing of skin irritations, rashes, and eczema symptoms. While chamomile can be found in capsule and liquid tincture form, it is commonly prepared as a tea using the dried flowers. If you have an allergy to ragweed, you may want to avoid chamomile because it is in the same botanical family.

Essential Oils

Leos like to express their individuality, and using fragrant essential oils as perfume is one way to do so.

NEROLI (*CITRUS AURANTIUM*)

Neroli is derived from the flower blossom of the Seville orange tree. Like the sign of Leo, neroli is associated with nobility, named after the seventeenth-century princess who first made it popular. This regal oil—with its sweetly floral scent—makes a wonderful perfume. Its fragrance is very calming, helping to inspire joy and banish restlessness. It's also said to have cooling properties and is therefore used for conditions of excess heat, including high blood pressure. You can soak in neroli's aromatic essence by sprinkling some in a hot bath. Or, dab a few drops on your heart and wear as a perfume. It can also be added to body lotion for enhancing circulation.

LEMON (*CITRUS LIMON*)

Like a Leo, lemon essential oil is bright, cheery, and makes people smile. The happiness elicited by lemon isn't solely due to its uplifting fragrance, but also because of the many benefits it provides. Lemon essential oil adds shine to the hair, cleanses

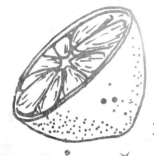

the scalp, improves sluggish circulation, and helps purify the air. Use lemon oil in a diffuser to lend an incandescent energy to a room. Lemon-scented body oil is uplifting and refreshing. Don't apply lemon oil straight to the skin, especially if you will be in the sun, as it can cause photosensitivity.

GERMAN CHAMOMILE (*MATRICARIA RECUTITA*)

German chamomile is a powerful example of the transformative energy of fire, the element that inspires the Leonine spirit; the heat used to distill the oil from the flower creates a new compound, chamazulene, well known for its anti-inflammatory properties and deep blue color. German chamomile is used to alleviate red, dry, and irritated skin. Its apple-like floral scent is soothing yet uplifting. You can add some German chamomile to a clay face mask to unmask your skin's true radiance. A few drops in a warm bath or used as a perfume will inspire a sunny and peaceful mood. Avoid German chamomile if you have an allergy to ragweed, as you'll likely be sensitive to it as well.

 # Flower Essences

Flower essences are created by placing blossoms in water and having the heat of the Sun, that which nourishes the Leo's spirit, alchemically draw out the flower's healing energies into the liquid. (See page 20 for how to use flower essences.)

BORAGE (*BORAGO OFFICINALIS*)

The quest of Leos is to live through their hearts, expressing warmth and love to themselves and those around them. Sometimes, though, being openhearted can be challenging; for example, it's hard to be emotionally buoyant when sadness and grief rest heavy in your heart. If you want some help in fortifying your courage, especially when feeling disheartened, try Borage flower essence.

INDIAN PAINTBRUSH (*CASTILLEJA MINIATA*)

With your sign representing self-expression, Leos are known as very creative people. You like artistic activities that allow you to show the world who you are and to be admired for the talents you embody. Yet, if you're like most people, you may experience times when your energy feels stuck and your creative juices are blocked. Indian Paintbrush flower essence can replenish your energy so that your imaginative visions can more readily manifest.

SUNFLOWER (*HELIANTHUS ANNUUS*)

With the Sun ruling Leo, you have a powerful ability to radiate your luminous essence into the world. Harnessing that inner solar fire requires a harmonious alliance with your masculine side, the part of your personality that helps you assert yourself and feel confident. Without this connection, low self-esteem or heightened self-glory can manifest, dimming the brilliance of your powerful self-expression. Sunflower flower essence can help bolster your solar energy, allowing your warmth and light to flourish.

 # Yoga Poses

Yoga can help Leos circulate radiant heat and energy throughout their bodies. Poses that focus on the heart, circulatory system, and spine can be particularly beneficial.

LION (*SIMHASANA*)

Lion pose will help you embody the inherent courage and fearlessness that reside in every Leo's heart. This playful posture encourages self-expression while it exercises your throat and eyes.

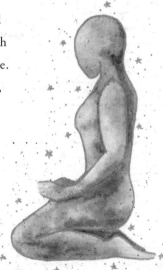

- Sit tall in a chair or on the floor. With your fingers spread wide, place your open palms on your knees. Inhale through your nose and exhale through your mouth, opening it wide. Stick out your tongue, reaching it down toward your chin, and loudly make the roaring sound "ha." Simultaneously, look up and lightly focus your eyes above the bridge of your nose. Repeat several times.

CAT (*MARJARYASANA*)

Another feline-inspired posture is Cat, which gently opens up your middle back and creates more space for your heart. It helps warm up the spine and massages your digestive organs without creating excess heat.

■ Place your hands and knees on the floor in tabletop position (your knees should align directly below your hips, with your elbows and wrists below your shoulders). Your neck should be in a neutral position with your eyes gazing toward the floor. Exhale, and while keeping your shoulders and knees in position, round your back toward the ceiling. Release your head between your arms so the crown of your head points toward the floor. Hold for several seconds, as you spread your shoulder blades wide across your upper back. Inhale, moving your spine back to tabletop position for several seconds. Repeat the sequence eight to twelve times.

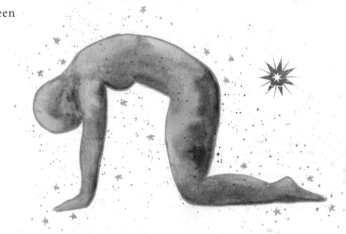

SPHINX (*SALAMBA BHUJANGASANA*)

In ancient Egypt, the sphinx—the mythological lion-bodied creature—was heralded as the temple guardian. Practicing the chest-opening Sphinx pose can help safeguard your very own temple—that of your heart.

■ Lie face down on your mat, with your feet hip-width apart and the tops of your feet touching the floor. Focus on keeping your legs grounded into the mat by pressing down through your pinky toe and lengthening out through your feet. Place your elbows directly under your shoulders, with your arms resting on the mat straight in front of you and your fingers spread wide. Push down through your forearms so your

Inspiring Sleep

Prize good sleep not only for the renewal it offers but that it will also lead to inspiring dreams, which may be key to enhancing your Leonine artistry. After all, they've had that effect for notable artists like Paul McCartney, Jasper Johns, and Mary Shelley, who discovered ideas for their opuses in their night-time journeys. If you're trying to work through a creative problem, practice dream incubation (see page 238). Before you go to sleep, ask your dreams to provide you with a sought-after solution to something that's been eluding you.

torso lifts into a mini backbend. Relax your shoulder blades down your back. Focus on lengthening your spine; gently engage your abdominal muscles to avoid compressing your lower back.

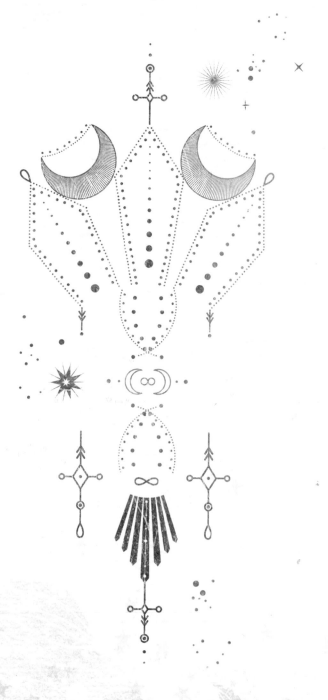

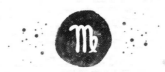

VIRGO

CHARACTERISTICS

Analytical, anxious, critical, detailed, diligent, efficient, helpful, logical, orderly, precise, rational, tidy.

SYMBOL

The Virgin, a symbol of purity and self-sufficiency. She is often depicted as a maiden holding a sheaf of grain, representing her association with fertility and the harvest. In mythological and cultural traditions, the Virgin is a symbol of sacred commitment, martyrdom, and the priestesses who tend the eternal flame.

PLANETARY RULER

Mercury, which has the fastest orbit around the Sun. Mercury was known for his role as the messenger of the gods. His counterpart in Greek mythology was Hermes. In astrology, Mercury represents the mind, communication, and language.

ELEMENT

Earth, which embodies the grounded energy of creativity, resistance, and practicality. It is fertile and passive, and it relates to the world on a sensual level. Pragmatism, routines, and sensuality energizes earth signs while fast movement, quick change, and an emphasis on sentimentality may deplete their vitality.

MODALITY

Mutable, which has an affinity for the adjustment and finessing stage of a creative project. Mutable signs are flexible, adaptive, and chameleon-like. They may find themselves agitated if things are too structured or overly defined.

Personal Health Profile

Virgo is associated with health consciousness, with people born under this sign diligently focused on being well and staying well. Yet, since Virgos are perfectionists, your idea of wellness may be a bit more exacting than others (after all, yours is the sign of the Virgin, making purity an enduring Virgoan goal). While someone else may accept a little ache or pain as one of life's trifles, not you. Detail-oriented Virgos are hyperaware of all their body's signs and signals; if anything seems even slightly amiss, you notice it and want to remedy it. Your analytical mind and fix-it nature spring into action, seeking a solution to the problem so that you can readily restore your sense of well-being.

While your keen sense of analysis and your critical eye may help you solve many health-care problems, these traits may, at times, also exacerbate them; after all, your vigilance about your body, combined with your unswerving desire to have everything just right, can lead to undue worry. As your mind and body are particularly in sync, the resulting anxiety may not only impact your mental outlook but also disturb your physical health. It's important for a Virgo to understand that in health, as in life, perfection is an unrealistic goal; it's not that you can't achieve it—it's that it just can't be achieved. Striving toward a more accepting outlook that allows for the existence of imperfections can do wonders for your sense of well-being and, ultimately, your physical health.

As the earth sign associated with the harvest, an important part of a Virgo's wellness regimen is centered on diet. Since your sign appreciates the bounty of the land, the joys and health benefits of organic and natural foods are probably nothing new to you.

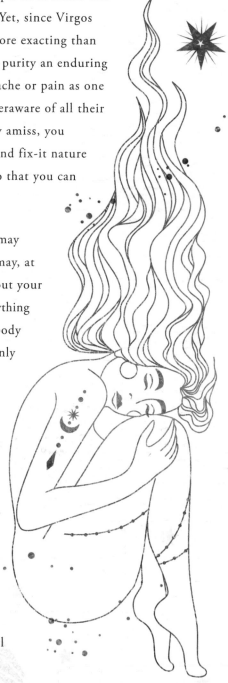

Your ideal health-care practitioner understands the inextricable link between mind and body. Whatever their scope of practice, you want them to be masters of their craft. Ideally, they are able to communicate both general concepts and details of health maintenance; this way, you can better understand how their recommendations fit together as practical steps for your attainment of optimal well-being.

 ## Areas of Health Focus

The parts of the body associated with Virgo include:

- The **small intestine**, an organ of digestion that absorbs many nutrients

- The **pancreas**, which produces digestive enzymes

- The **gallbladder**, which stores bile, necessary to break down fats

Your Virgoan critical-thinking skills, keen physical awareness, and perceptive mind are some of the resources you can use when facing any health challenge.

AID DIGESTION

Discern and *assimilate* are two key words used to describe Virgo as well as the function of the small intestine, an organ ruled by your sign. As such, Virgos may want to pay careful attention to their digestive health. Excess stress and the routine intake of aspirin and other nonsteroidal anti-inflammatory drugs (NSAIDs) can lead to intestinal permeability, a cause of indigestion and nutrient malabsorption. One way to boost intestinal health is to eat a diet rich in anti-inflammatory nutrients, including omega-3 fatty acids (featured in cold-water fish) as well as the flavonoid and carotenoid phytonutrients found concentrated in richly colored fruits and vegetables. Probiotic supplements can also be helpful, as they promote the reestablishment of healthy populations of beneficial intestinal flora.

RESPECT FOOD SENSITIVITIES

Virgos are very discriminating: your methodical nature compels you to discern the good from the not-so-good. Combine this with the fact that your sign governs the act of digestion, and you've got a recipe for food sensitivities. In this physiological event, your body readily judges foods as either friend or foe, with the latter triggering inflammation that can lead to nutrient malabsorption. Food sensitivities can also cause indigestion, depression, and headaches. If these symptoms are on your list of health complaints and the causes remain an undiagnosed mystery, you may want to investigate the possibility of adverse food reactions with your health-care practitioner.

PROMOTE GALLBLADDER HEALTH

Traditional Chinese medicine—fond of describing the body in poetic ways—portrays the gallbladder as exacting and decisive, characteristics that also describe your sign. The gallbladder serves as a storehouse for bile. Without adequate bile, fats aren't well digested, which can lead to malabsorption and food sensitivities. The Western diet, filled with refined foods and overloaded with saturated fats, exacerbates gallbladder disturbances. As fiber-filled whole foods promote the health of this small—but very important—organ, include a cornucopia of fruits, vegetables, whole grains, and other nutrient-rich fare in your diet.

PRACTICE ACCEPTANCE

Virgos are quite proficient at dissecting situations—analyzing the ins and outs of all the details. While your critical mind provides you with astonishing insights, it can also lead to an amazing amount of worry owing to your perfectionist proclivity to readily view that things just aren't the best that they can be. It's important to remember that not every situation needs remedying. Learning to accept situations and people (including yourself) just as they are, with flaws and all, will reduce your stress and enhance your mental and physical health.

 # Healthy Eating Tips

As Virgo is an earth sign, those born under it have an instinctive knowledge that food can play an integral role in maintaining well-being. In fact, you were probably into "health food" long before it became a trend, let alone more mainstream.

AVOID FOOD TRIGGERS

Do you sense that certain foods may trigger feelings of malaise—whether they be digestive upsets or unsettling mood swings? If so, consider doing a modified allergy-avoidance or full-scale elimination diet to determine whether any foods you eat deplete your vitality. Even just eliminating the food-trigger triple threat—wheat, cow's milk, and eggs—from your diet for two weeks may do wonders for wellness and allow you to deduce whether you are sensitive to one or more of these common food allergens. For a more detailed and methodical approach, consider pursuing an elimination diet with the guidance of a nutritionist.

THINK GLOBALLY, EAT LOCALLY

With yours being the sign of the harvest, Virgos are naturally connected to, and concerned about, the Earth. Empower yourself by purchasing locally grown and organic foods. Doing so can make a different in the sustainability of the environment and your health, as organic foods are lower in pesticide residues than conventionally grown foods. By shopping at farmers' markets, you'll not only enjoy the freshest produce, meats, and dairy products, but you'll also directly support the people who grow the foods that nourish you. Look for foods that are labeled organic, but don't discount the wares of local farmers who may grow their food sustainably but who have decided not to incur the extra expense of getting their farms organically certified.

WATCH OBSESSIVE EATING PATTERNS

Health-oriented Virgos may want to keep their tendency toward austerity and their affection for details in check. Otherwise, you may find yourself developing orthorexic habits. The term *orthorexia* signifies an obsession with the ideas of healthy eating, where a good portion of your energy is spent worrying about which foods to eat and how they will impact your health. This often occurs at the expense of life balance, the enjoyment of food, and, ironically, optimal health. If you find yourself following a supposedly healthy diet that leaves you low in energy or feeling isolated, you may want to consider whether it is really the best plan for your well-being.

 # Health-Supporting Foods

Strongly connected to the land, Virgos appreciate the bounty that nature yields. Whole grains, bitter greens, and the macrobiotic staple umeboshi plums are some of the many natural foods that may support a Virgo's health.

WHOLE GRAINS

The symbol for your sign, the Virgin, is often depicted holding a sheaf of grain, a food that can play a health-promoting role in a Virgo's diet. Yet it's important to use your discriminating nature when selecting which grains to enjoy. Fiber-rich whole grains are better for you than ones that have been refined, which are stripped of many of their naturally occurring nutrients. While wheat is ubiquitous in the Western diet, you may want to avoid it as your sole go-to grain because it's a top food allergen. Instead, enjoy a cornucopia of whole grains such as barley, spelt, teff, and quinoa; the latter two are great for people who are also gluten reactive.

BITTER GREENS

According to Chinese medicine, bitter flavors enhance the function of the Virgo-ruled small intestine, making bitter greens—such as dandelion greens, sorrel, and endive—a sweet addition to a Virgo's healthful diet. These vegetables aid digestion, as their bitter compounds stimulate secretion of hydrochloric acid, digestive enzymes, and bile; the fact that they are rich in fiber is an added plus. You can use bitter greens as a basis for a dinner salad. Also, try a splash of bitters, the bar condiment made from gentian and other herbs, in sparkling water for a delicious digestion-aiding aperitif.

UMEBOSHI PLUMS

Efficient Virgos will find much to love in umeboshi plums, as this food has so many health benefits. Made from pickled ume plums, this Japanese alkalizing wonder is said to curb indigestion and enhance mineral absorption, while also having a stellar reputation as a hangover remedy. Combined with well-cooked rice, it is part of a traditional Japanese recipe given to children when they're sick. It is available as whole plums, pureed paste, or vinegar. You can find it in natural food stores and Asian markets. With its tart-salty flavor, umeboshi plums can adorn steamed vegetables or add a zing to rice dishes. It's also combined with perilla leaves to make the delicious ume-shiso sushi roll.

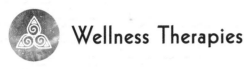

Wellness Therapies

Wellness therapies that promote detoxification can offer you numerous healing rewards, allowing you to cleanse your body in pursuit of the purity that Virgos so cherish.

FASTING

For Virgos, a little sacrifice is a small price to pay for the reward of purity. Fasting reflects these ascetic aims by restricting your intake of food and cleansing the body of unwanted toxins. While water-only fasts are used therapeutically for a host of different conditions, a less restrictive approach to consider is a modified juice fast, which can also incorporate broths, fruits, and steamed vegetables. While many spas offer supervised fasting programs, you can also choose to do one at home under the guidance of a nutrition practitioner. Fastidious Virgos should remember that fasting may be beneficial when done periodically, but fasting too often may not be health supportive.

STEAM BATHS

Traditional steam baths—such as the Russian *banya*—offer an ordered and ritualized approach to cleansing, an attribute that is certain to attract health-conscious Virgos. At a banya, you alternate between sweating out toxins in a sultry steam room and cooling off by plunging into a cold pool. The heat brings blood to your skin while the cold water sends the flow of blood inward to nourish your organs. Yet, steam baths are not limited to the Russian culture; if there's no banya in your area, see if there's a Korean *jjimjilbang* or Turkish *hamam*. Or create your own bathing ritual at the gym, alternating between the steam room and a cold shower.

HERBAL WRAPS

Herbal wraps are perfect for earthy Virgos looking for a relaxing approach to detoxification. During this treatment you're swathed in herb-infused linens. The heat created by this cocooning as well as the herbs' stimulating effects help your body release toxins. After being unwrapped, you are rinsed off and a moisturizing lotion is applied to further soften your skin. If you're prone to feelings of claustrophobia, opt to keep your arms outside of the sheets. Also, ask which herbs are used in the treatment to ensure they are not ones to which you are sensitive.

Relaxation Practices

Relaxation practices can help Virgos quiet their minds, which are often sowed with worry and concern, giving them the freedom to feel at ease.

CRAFTING

With an eye for detail and an appreciation for functional aesthetics, Virgos are the craftspeople of the zodiac. Channel and express your inner artisan—crochet scarves, design mosaic garden tiles, refinish your bookcase, or do some other DIY activity. You can explore endless craft project possibilities that allow you to flex your creative muscle and relax your mind. With crafting having experienced a renaissance, there are many resources—magazines, websites, and classes—from which you can learn new skills. If your creations meet with kudos from friends and family, consider turning your hobby into a side business. And, as with all your endeavors, try to temper your inner critic: instead, revel in appreciation of the unique wares you create.

GARDENING

Planting a garden and enjoying the fruits—and vegetables—of your labor can be a deliciously enriching and rewarding experience. If you don't have a yard, you can still exercise your green thumb by growing an indoor herb garden. Pots of sage, mint, and oregano will not only brighten your kitchen but will also add splendor to your recipes. If you are new to gardening, or just need a refresher, contact the Master Gardeners in your area. This community-oriented service features local volunteers who can provide you with practical tips on sustainable gardening practices.

ANIMAL COMPANIONSHIP

Spending time with a dog or cat is a great antidote for stress, especially for a Virgo; after all, astrologically speaking, your sign is associated with pets. Not only do pets happily lap up the attention you give them, but you also get something deeply nourishing for your sensitive soul in return—their healing, unconditional love. Consider volunteering at your local animal shelter, spending time playing with puppies, or fostering rescued kittens. You get to enjoy the animals while you also get to enjoy the rewards of doing a good deed.

Natural Remedies

Since yours is an earth sign, Virgos appreciate the benefit of using natural-based substances, such as herbs and dietary supplements, to promote their well-being.

VALERIAN (*VALERIANA OFFICINALIS*)

Valerian has long been associated with Mercury, Virgo's ruling planet. This connection makes sense given that worry-prone Virgos may benefit from this nerve-relaxing herb. Research studies have found that valerian may be helpful as a natural sleep aid, inducing a sense of calm that allows you to fall asleep more quickly. Unlike pharmaceutical drugs used for this purpose, valerian is nonaddictive and won't make you groggy the next morning. Yet, while valerian offers great benefits, it has a rather off-putting smell. Consequently, valerian tea may not be the best approach; opt instead for capsules or tinctures. Valerian is often featured with other sedative herbs such as lemon balm, passionflower, and skullcap in combination herbal products.

DIGESTIVE ENZYMES

When the Virgo-ruled small intestine has inadequate amounts of digestive enzymes—whether as a result of aging or eating a refined-food diet—fats, carbohydrates, and protein cannot be broken down effectively. This reduces the amount of energy you get from your food and can also lead to digestive difficulties such as bloating, gas, and heartburn. Enzyme dietary supplements can help replenish your own internal enzyme supplies, aiding in healthy digestion. Many digestive enzyme supplements are plant-based, usually extracted from pineapple or papaya, or from Aspergillus fungus. Yet, vegetarians may want to read the labels closely as some supplements are actually derived from animal pancreases.

MULTIVITAMIN SUPPLEMENTS

Virgos take a holistic approach to life and like to cover all their bases. So consider taking a high-quality multivitamin supplement to secure the range of your nutritional needs.

While not a substitute for a healthy diet, a multivitamin can be an important adjunct that ensures you're getting optimal nutrition. Although they're generally called multivitamins, most also contain a gamut of minerals and other nutrients as well. These supplements come in multiple forms—for example, some formulas are food-based while others are synthetically derived—so read the labels to determine which are the best for you. With a multivitamin, like with everything, you get what you pay for, so spend a little more for a high-quality supplement.

 ## Essential Oils

Since Virgos appreciate the parts that comprise the whole, they are sure to be drawn to aromatherapy, the art of distilling fragrant essential oils from flowers, herbs, and fruits.

MELISSA (*MELISSA OFFICINALIS*)

Melissa and Virgos have many things in common, not the least of which is that both are renowned for their virtues. Throughout history, sweet-smelling melissa—also known as lemon balm—has been lauded for its many merits, including its antiviral activity and its ability to reduce anxiety and melancholy. When your worries have you up late at night, a melissa-infused hot bath may help allay a tendency toward insomnia. Grow a pot of lemon balm, from which you can make a delightfully calming tea. When it comes to choosing a melissa oil, don't skimp on quality; cheaper products are often adulterated with citronella and lemongrass oils, and don't feature the same benefits that pure melissa oil provides.

CARDAMOM (*ELETTARIA CARDAMOMUM*)

Cardamom essential oil is derived from the pungent and aromatic spice of the same name, widely used in Indian cuisine. Cardamom oil's warm fragrance is calming yet uplifting, and it has been used in perfume blends dating back to ancient Egypt. Well known for its aphrodisiac properties, cardamom essential oil can help disrobe the Virgoan modesty that may camouflage your sexual fire. You can add a few drops of cardamom oil to unscented body lotion and use in a sensuality-inspired massage. A tea made from boiled cardamom seeds mixed with honey will not only relax your mind but will also calm an upset stomach.

CARROT SEED (*DAUCUS CAROTA*)

Carrot seed oil is distilled from the seed of this root vegetable, governed by Mercury, your planetary ruler. It is a great addition to a skin-care regimen, as it is prized for its softening and rejuvenating qualities. Its liver-supporting and diuretic properties make it a great adjunct for detoxifying, a benefit certain to be appreciated by the health-conscious Virgo. You can enliven your skin by mixing carrot seed oil into your moisturizer and body lotion, or add the oil to a clay mask to enhance its soothing and cleansing properties. Enjoy the detoxifying attributes, as well as earthy sweet fragrance, of carrot seed oil by adding a few drops to your bath.

 # Flower Essences

Earth-centered Virgos are sure to be intrigued by flower essences, elixirs of the Earth that help balance emotional and psychological well-being. (See page 20 for how to use flower essences.)

PINE (*PINUS SYLVESTRIS*)

Virgos hold everything—most notably themselves—to very high standards. Consequently, as a perfectionist, you may be haunted with self-reproach when a situation doesn't yield the outcome you intended. You may view this lack of success as a reflection of personal failure, taking up the mantle of blame, even if it was a situation over which you really had little—if any—control. Pine is a great flower essence to help you release self-deprecating feelings and realize that the perfection you should strive for is complete and unconditional self-acceptance.

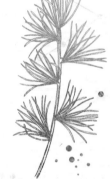

CENTAURY (*CENTAURIUM UMBELLATUM*)

Being of service is the raison d'être for Virgos, a virtue that has become your calling card. With friends, family, and coworkers clamoring for your advice, assistance, and time, it's often challenging for a Virgo to know when to say *no*. Centaury flower essence can help you draw boundaries, gracefully maintaining your giving and dedicated nature without feeling encumbered by the needs of those around you. It can help you realize that saying no is sometimes as healing for you, and others, as saying *yes*.

ROCK WATER

Efficient Virgos like to organize themselves by way of schedules, routines, and systems, with order bringing them a sense of comfort. While this ritualized approach to life can make you more productive, it can also hamper your spontaneity, which is an important ingredient of joy and creativity. Rock Water flower essence allows you to engage the energy of the two elements represented in its name: the solidity of the rock combined with the fluid energy of water.

 # Yoga Poses

Yoga provides Virgos with another way to connect with their bodies and minds. Practicing yoga requires concentration as well as attention to detail, both traits for which Virgos are well known.

SEATED FORWARD BEND (*PASCHIMOTTANASANA*)

While this seated posture seems simple, it provides a mindful experience of being present as you fold onto yourself. It helps calm anxiousness and the overanalytical Virgoan mind while toning the digestive organs.

■ Sit on the floor with your legs extended straight in front of you. Adjust your buttocks so that your sit bones are on the floor. Without locking your knees, activate your legs by pushing your thighs into the floor and extending out through your flexed feet. Inhale and lengthen your torso, and then slowly bend forward at the hips. Grab the sides of your feet, or shins, with your hands (or use a strap around your feet if your hamstrings feel tight). Point your gaze toward your toes. With each inhalation, lengthen your torso, and see if you can naturally go deeper into the bend. Stay in the pose for up to two minutes. (If, as you bend forward, your back isn't straight, consider sitting on a folded blanket or bending your knees.)

HALF LORD OF THE FISHES (*ARDHA MATSYENDRASANA*)

This seated spinal twist massages the intestines and
stimulates digestion. During a twist, you spiral around
your central core—your spine—catalyzing a freer flow
of energy throughout the body as well as the mind.

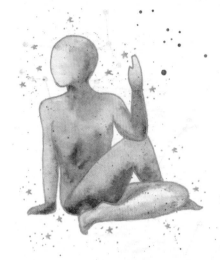

- Sit on the floor with your legs extended straight
  in front of you. Adjust your buttocks so that
  your sit bones are on the floor. Bend your knees
  and place your feet on the floor in front of you.
  Slide your right foot under your left leg until
  your right foot is near your left hip and your
  right thigh is pointing straight out in front of you.
  Then place your left foot on the outside of your right thigh (your left knee should
  point up to the ceiling). Sit tall, exhale, and then twist to the left, drawing your belly
  in toward your spine. Place your left hand on the floor behind your left buttock, and
  either wrap your right arm around your left knee or place your right elbow on the
  outside on your left leg near your knee. Turn your head either in the direction of the
  twist or in the opposite direction. Stay in the pose for up to one minute.

EXTENDED PUPPY (*UTTANA SHISHOSANA*)

With your sign governing pets, why not pay homage to one with your yoga practice?
Extended Puppy pose gently stretches your spine while relaxing your mind. It's a calming
posture to do before sleep to help ward off insomnia.

- Place your hands and knees on the floor in
  tabletop position (your knees should
  align directly below your hips,
  with your elbows and wrists
  below your shoulders). Curl
  your toes under and extend
  your arms straight out
  in front of you,

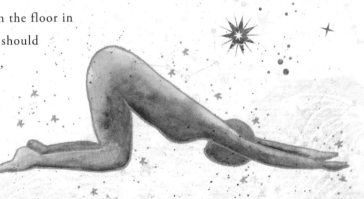

keeping them long and strong. Move your buttocks back in the direction of your heels, lengthening your spine and stretching your lower back. Rest your forehead on the floor or on a yoga block. Hold the posture for up to one minute. To come out of the pose, gently sit back on your heels.

Inspiring Sleep

Virgos are keenly attuned to details and love things to be organized. As you prize order, disorder in your bedroom may impede your feeling at ease. A cluttered space may mirror itself in a mind that feels restless and filled with disquietude, readily keeping you from drifting off to sleep. Keeping your bedroom clean and applying feng shui principles (see page 112) so that the energy in the room flows more seamlessly can transform your bedroom into a sleep and dream sanctuary.

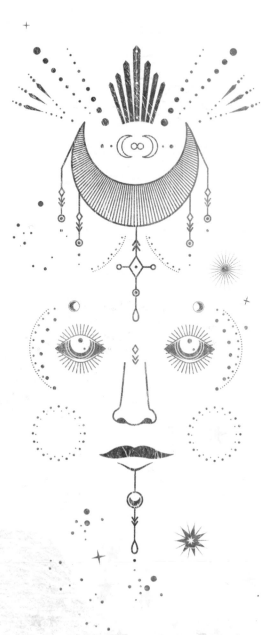

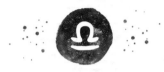

LIBRA

CHARACTERISTICS

Charming, diplomatic, equitable, gracious, indecisive, judicious, orderly, poised, romantic, sociable, stylish, sybaritic.

SYMBOL

The Scales, a symbol of justice, balance, and equality. Reflective of Libra's association with measurement and value, the *libra* was the basic unit of weight in ancient Rome. In mythological and cultural traditions, the Scales are a symbol of law, truth, and morality.

PLANETARY RULER

Venus, the brightest planet in the solar system. Venus was the Roman goddess of beauty and love, who represented sexuality, pleasure, and fertility. Her counterpart in Greek mythology was Aphrodite. In astrology, Venus represents love, beauty, and the force of attraction.

ELEMENT

Air, which is associated with the agile energy of thoughts, observation, and logic. It is social, intellectual, changeable, and relationship oriented. Mental activities, communicating, and creating alliances energizes air signs while stasis, too much practicality, and heightened emotionality may deplete their vitality.

MODALITY

Cardinal, which loves beginnings and the first stage of a creative project. Cardinal signs are motivated, ambitious, and enterprising. They encounter stress when things are not fresh and new.

Personal Health Profile

Libras dislike when things are out of balance, including their health. Since you appreciate the beauty of harmony, any physical sign or symptom that leaves you feeling less than peaceful—even one that would be perceived as inconsequential to most—registers strongly on the Libran wellness scale.

When you do feel off-kilter, you'll work hard to find resolution to your problems and negotiate your way back to health. To do so, Libras often seek the advice of their large social networks—friends and acquaintances alike—to find the most respected health-care practitioners to help restore their physical equipoise. As you place a good deal of faith in the power of relationships, you're likely to find it more gratifying and effective to work with a health advocate than travel the wellness path solo.

Yet, Libras are not quick to make decisions regarding their health care (or much else, for that matter). With the Scales as your astrological totem, a sharp-minded Libra will weigh all the pros and cons of various options—seeking second and sometimes third options whenever possible. While this judicious approach to decision making often results in very satisfying and beneficial outcomes, be careful that it doesn't lead to excessive procrastination, a Libran pitfall.

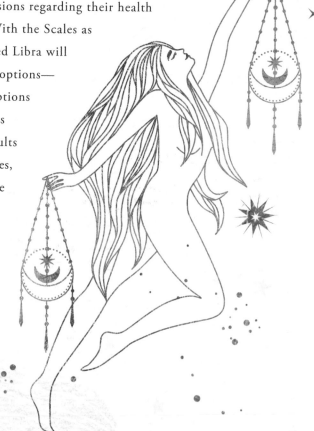

While those born under the sign of the Scales may seem outwardly calm and collected, Libras tend to carry around their fair share of stress, a result of the agitation they experience when faced with disagreeable situations. While disinclined to overtly express your woes (thinking it too brash for your refined Libran sensibilities), your disquietude may instead be expressed in your body, notably in the Libra-associated lower back, kidneys, and skin.

Libras will be more motivated to be active in their wellness journeys if they involve activities that are luxurious, pleasurable, and refined, characteristics that speak fluently to your sybaritic nature. For example, Libras will favor a weight-loss diet that allows a daily dose of wine and chocolate over one that requires ascetic sacrifice. Reflecting your cooperative and social nature, finding a workout partner or inviting a friend to join you at the day spa will help you stay more interested and engaged in your personal wellness program.

 ## Areas of Health Focus

The parts of the body associated with Libra include:

- The **lumbar region**, the vertebrae in your lower back, which helps you stand tall

- The **islets of Langerhans**, a group of pancreatic cells that synthesize blood sugar-regulating insulin

- The **kidneys**, which are balanced on either side of your spine and are responsible for maintaining homeostasis

- The **skin**, the organ that sheathes your body and serves as an interface with the environment

Your Libran resilient will, solution-seeking mind, and need for harmony are some of the resources you can use when facing any health challenge.

BACK UP BACK HEALTH

In the name of peace and harmony, Libras tend to bend over backward for others. While your gracious and accommodating disposition is second nature, it isn't without its stress, which may take refuge in the Libra-ruled lower back, translating to pain and stiffness. Chiropractic, massage, and acupuncture (see page 167) can be beneficial in promoting back health, as can graceful, yet strengthening, fitness approaches such as Pilates and Gyrotonics.

Ensuring your workspace has good ergonomics and your mattress is adequately supportive can also be helpful, whether you have a bad back or just want to prevent one. Also, when shopping for shoes, consider function as well as fashion; unsupportive shoes—including those stylish high heels that Libras love to wear—can throw your back out of whack.

MAINTAIN BLOOD SUGAR BALANCE

The innate Libran temperament is one of equilibrium. Yet with your sign's planetary ruler, Venus, associated with blood sugar, balance may not come as naturally to your glucose levels. While there can be a genetic component to developing blood sugar imbalances, lifestyle factors are just as important, making this area of your health one in which you can exert a good level of control. Maintaining optimal weight and switching to a whole foods diet are important for keeping blood sugar in check. A regular fitness routine is beneficial, too, as exercise improves your cells' sensitivity to insulin, which helps maintain glucose balance.

SUPPORT YOUR KIDNEYS

In pure Libran fashion, the role of the kidneys—ruled by your sign—involves maintaining balance, keeping our internal environment in the steady state required for it to function properly; it does this through such vital functions as ridding the body of waste, excess water, and surplus electrolytes. Diabetes and hypertension can impinge on kidney health, as can smoking. Drinking six to eight glasses of water each day is important for keeping the kidneys—and the rest of the body—in tip-top shape. In traditional Chinese medicine, it is said that the kidneys are negatively affected by fear; therefore, working on feeling more empowered may do wonders for the health of these organs, let alone your general well-being.

ENHANCE SKIN HEALTH

Libras love all things refined, including physical beauty, which is one reason they pay attention to, and take pride in, their appearance. So the fact that natives of your sign experience skin issues—including breakouts—may seem like a cruel irony. You can do many things to promote skin health and put your "best face" forward: watch that Libran tendency to overindulge in sweets and alcohol; help your kidneys flush out toxins by keeping yourself well hydrated; and take the time to follow a thorough skin-care regimen, including regular cleansing, exfoliating, moisturizing, and sun protection.

Healthy Eating Tips

Being sociable, Libras enjoy numerous opportunities to enjoy delicious meals in the company of others. While this can bring you pleasure, it can also pose a challenge to sticking to a healthy-eating plan.

EAT FOR BLOOD SUGAR BALANCE

If you want to keep your blood sugar balanced, consider some simple dietary strategies. Eat whole foods, such as vegetables, fruits, beans, and whole grains, which are rich in fiber and antioxidants. Also, cut down on refined sugars, processed carbohydrates, and animal protein, excesses of which can increase diabetes risk. Eating several small meals throughout the day, rather than larger ones spaced far apart, can help keep glucose levels balanced. You can further refine a blood sugar-balancing diet by favoring foods with a low glycemic index (GI); these are ones whose carbohydrates break down more slowly and therefore don't lead to rapid elevations of blood sugar.

INFUSE MEALS WITH GRACIOUSNESS

Artistic Libras have an inherent need for aesthetic fulfillment, and beauty around you nurtures a sense of peace within. Take this into consideration when preparing meals by turning them into small works of art. This will enhance your enjoyment of food and make meals even more soulfully nourishing. You can do this by making each dining experience one of artistic beauty. Pretty plates and serving pieces can add grandeur to even the simplest of meals. Use candles, place mats, and cloth napkins to further enhance the elegance of your meal (regardless of whether it's a four-course feast with friends or take-out Thai on your own).

TRUST YOUR GUT

Libras have a propensity for indecision that can extend to their ability to make food choices. Even the smallest of considerations can seem monumental at the time. This is especially true when you're in the company of others, compounding your dilemma; after all, you care what other people think of you and don't want to make the "wrong choice." To know what's best for you in the moment, including what foods will be the most nourishing, tune into your inner voice during mealtimes. Don't forget that oftentimes there is no one best option, but equally good selections; remembering this can help release the flood of decision-making pressure you may feel when ordering.

 # Health-Supporting Foods

As Libras always want to strike a balance, it's nice to know that there are many foods that can provide you with both pleasure and health-promoting benefits. Foods associated with your planetary ruler, Venus, that support Libran health include berries, beans, and artichokes.

BERRIES

Brimming with nutrients, especially phytonutrients with anticancer and anti-inflammatory properties, berries can spruce up your health. Raspberries and blackberries are especially rich in fiber, while many people drink cranberry juice as prevention for urinary tract infections. Venus-ruled berries are considered a low- to medium-glycemic-index food and therefore won't elevate blood sugar as much as many other fruits. You can enjoy berries in smoothies, salads, and a range of delicious desserts, from cobblers to fruit salads. Making homemade berry jam can be a satisfying, let alone nutrient-rich, activity. If fresh berries aren't readily accessible, buy frozen ones.

BEANS

Looking to keep your blood sugar on an even keel? Enjoy more beans. High in fiber and protein, and low on the glycemic index, these little treasures help balance glucose levels and may reduce the risk of developing diabetes. Whether they are black, kidney, navy, or garbanzo, beans are always a great addition to your meal plan. To reduce their cooking time and enhance their digestibility, presoak your beans. Place them in a bowl, cover them with water, and keep the bowl in a cool place or the refrigerator for at least eight hours. Both cooking time and water amount vary depending upon bean type; you can readily access charts that detail both either online or in cookbooks.

ARTICHOKES

It's no surprise that artichokes are another Venus-ruled food. After all, even the process of eating one is sensual, as are the taste and texture of its delicate heart. This fact wasn't lost on the ancient Romans, who held artichokes in high esteem as aphrodisiacs. Yet these Venusian properties aren't all they provide—artichokes help you finely tune your health by offering good amounts of fiber, folic acid, and potassium. To cook an artichoke, first cut off the bottom stem so it is balanced while cooking. Remove the first few outer leaves, and trim a ½ inch (1 cm) off the top. Place in a steamer bowl and cook until the outer leaves readily pull away from the center, about twenty to forty minutes, depending upon size. Eat the heart and the bottom parts of the leaves, discarding the inner fibrous part.

 # Wellness Therapies

With the goddess of beauty ruling your sign, pampering treatments that help you look your best hold great value to a Libra's sense of wellness.

FACIALS

Even if beauty is only skin deep, it's still essential to take care of your skin. Facials can do wonders for making it glow and helping you feel beautiful inside and out. During a facial, your skin is exfoliated, deeply cleansed, and moisturized. You're also treated to a face and scalp massage that is not only sumptuous but also therapeutic, as it stimulates the lymphatic system to clear away impurities that may contribute to a less-than-radiant appearance. While professional facials can do wonders for your skin, don't forget the benefits of also doing them at home. To do so, gently wash your face, do a steam treatment and then some light exfoliation followed by a mask suited to your skin type.

SUGAR BODY POLISH

A sugar body polish is a great treatment for Libras who like everything, including their skin, to be smooth and refined. Not only does sugar's granular texture help slough off dead skin cells, but sugar also contains glycolic acid, which further adds to its exfoliating properties. Polished skin looks better and translates into better health because it can more readily absorb moisture and shed impurities. Products you can use for a DIY body polish treatment abound; look for ones that feature evaporated sugarcane juice rather than refined sugar. These scrubs often contain other ingredients—such as fruit and botanical extracts—added for their therapeutic and cosmetic properties.

LOMILOMI MASSAGE

To a Libra, relationships are works of art; like any masterpiece, they are deeply inspiring, satisfying, and healing. Lomilomi, a traditional Hawaiian massage practice, offers a Libra another way to benefit from relationships as this massage is often performed by not one but two practitioners. Working in unison, they rhythmically massage different parts of your body. In addition to relieving muscular tension, lomilomi does wonders for relieving mental tension. This massage style, often referred to as "loving hands," calls on gracefulness, dance-inspired movements, and intuition, qualities a Libra greatly appreciates.

 # Relaxation Practices

Libras are most peaceful when beauty and harmony surround them and when they feel free to express the inherent grace and artistry they naturally embrace.

FENG SHUI

As Libras are so sensitive to disharmony, if your environment isn't in order, it can make you feel "out of order." To enjoy a deeper sense of harmony, consider feng shui-ing your living and/or workspace. Feng shui—known as the Chinese art of placement—uses furniture positioning, color choice, and auspicious items (such as wind chimes) to unblock energetic disturbances in the environment that are thought to inhibit one's ability to acquire good fortune and achieve optimal health. Feng shui has become popular in the West, making it easy to find books and websites on the subject. If you don't want to learn the techniques yourself, you can always hire a trained practitioner to feng shui your space.

TAI CHI

Grace in action could as easily describe a Libra as it could tai chi. This martial arts form has gained popularity in the West as a serene approach to exercise and stress relief. Tai chi features slow, dancelike movements, with each pose flowing seamlessly into the next.

It's a moving meditation that provides the body with an opportunity to gain agility and strength. Although there are many books on tai chi available, learning from a qualified instructor in a class setting—whether in person or online—can provide you with the personalized, yet social, experience that Libras appreciate. Look for tai chi classes at community centers, health clubs, and colleges in your area.

WRITING POETRY

Libras are so concerned that their words or actions will cause discord that they often restrain their true self-expression. Therefore, it can be especially important to find supportive outlets, such as writing poetry, that give you freedom to openly articulate your creative mind. Aligned with your innate sense of grace, poetry honors words not only for their ability to express meaning but also for the aesthetic qualities they embody. Writing haikus, in particular, may be a good poetry practice for a Libra. These short poetic verses, composed of just three lines and seventeen syllables, can provide you with an opportunity to balance the desire for expressing meaning with the need to maintain a well-defined order.

 # Natural Remedies

Herbs, dietary supplements, and other natural remedies can do justice to a self-care regimen aimed at promoting optimal health.

FENUGREEK (*TRIGONELLA FOENUM-GRAECUM*)

Libras will enjoy fenugreek's beautifying properties. Mix ground seeds with water for calming skin irritations, or with some yogurt and use as a hair conditioner. One of fenugreek's traditional uses, helping those with diabetes, has been supported by studies that show it can lower blood sugar and total cholesterol levels. Traditional Chinese medicine also uses it for kidney ailments. Fenugreek is available as a supplement in capsule or liquid tincture form. You can find fenugreek seeds, which you can grind at home and use in recipes (it is a staple of curry blends), in the spice section of natural food stores and specialty food markets.

BURDOCK (*ARCTIUM LAPPA*)

Burdock is governed by your planetary ruler, Venus. And while with its rough-hewn appearance it may not have the elegance often associated with Venus, with its clinging burrs, it is tenacious, just like the mythic goddess herself. With its numerous benefits, it can clear up many health imbalances: it is known as a blood purifier, diuretic, and promoter of kidney health. This is likely why it has traditionally been used to help control breakouts and bolster the appearance of the skin. Burdock root is available in capsule or liquid tincture form. Fresh burdock root, found in Asian food markets, is also a commonly consumed therapeutic food in Japanese cuisine.

COLLAGEN PEPTIDES

One of the hallmarks of aging is the reduction in the body's production of collagen, a protein vital to the strength of our joints as well as the health of our skin. Recent research has suggested that collagen peptide supplements can increase skin hydration and elasticity. They are often found as ingredients in energy bars or as a powder that can be added to smoothies. Bone broths are another concentrated source. Collagen peptides—whether from supplements or broth—are derived from animals and therefore may not be of interest to vegetarians. Another way to help boost collagen production is through the adequate consumption of vitamin C and silica, two nutrients that play a role in supporting the body's synthesis of this skin-supportive protein.

 # Essential Oils

Aromatherapy offers Libras an exquisitely delightful way to experience wellness. Fragrant essential oils not only smell wonderful but can also be used cosmetically in creams and toners to enhance beauty.

DAMASK ROSE (*ROSA DAMASCENA*)

If there were one flower that is associated with the Venusian concepts of beauty and love, it would be the rose. In addition to featuring a heart-opening fragrance, oil made from the damask rose has radiant skin-enhancing properties. Remember, though: while a Libra may like the equanimity of the fair-minded sentiment "A rose is a rose is a rose," it doesn't actually hold true for different types of damask rose oils: rose otto and rose absolute have different qualities, owing to the former being produced by steam distillation and the latter through chemical solvents. Use damask rose as a perfume, or add it to your bathwater for a luxuriously romantic experience. As rose oil is very expensive (it takes thousands of pounds (kilograms) of petals to make 1 ounce (29 ml) of oil), it is often diluted with jojoba oil.

ROSE GERANIUM (*PELARGONIUM GRAVEOLENS*)

A cousin of the red-colored geraniums that adorn many windowsills, rose geranium is one of the premier skin-care oils. Like a Libra, it doesn't discriminate—it can create balance in either overly dry or oily skin. It is also an energizing pick-me-up, inspiring the mind and body when stress and fatigue drain your energy reserves. The scent of rose geranium is said to inspire relaxed spontaneity, helpful to Libras when they feel encumbered by indecision. For a skin-balancing toner, add some rose geranium oil to a mister bottle of water, or mix some oil into your favorite cleansing mask. With its warm and rosy scent, it also makes a lovely perfume.

PEPPERMINT (*MENTHA PIPERITA*)

Similar to Libra, which is known for its qualities of cordiality and graciousness, peppermint is symbol of hospitality. When your solution-searching mind needs a bit of a boost, you'll appreciate peppermint's ability to relieve mental fatigue and enhance concentration. It also has renowned stomach-soothing properties, making it a wonderful digestive aid, especially after a rich and heavy meal; for a delicious after-meal stomach settler, enjoy a cup of mint tea. You can add a little peppermint oil to your facial cleanser to help balance out any red or dry patches. The smell of mint is a refreshing way to start your day, giving your brain an early morning boost.

 # Flower Essences

That these healing elixirs are made from beautiful botanicals is one reason Libras will be attracted to flower essences. (See page 20 for how to use flower essences.)

SCLERANTHUS (*SCLERANTHUS ANNUUS*)

As the diplomats of the zodiac, Libras possess a deep-seated desire for mediating resolution.

Yet, while you are masterful at helping others make decisions, it is somewhat more challenging for Libras to do so in their own personal lives, owing to the fear that they'll choose wrongly or alienate others. When you find yourself with excessive wavering, in the throes of battling bouts of indecision and wanting to feel more connected to a calm sense of inner resolve, try Scleranthus flower essence.

SCARLET MONKEYFLOWER (*MIMULUS CARDINALIS*)

While Libras appear easygoing, with your heightened sensitivity to injustice, your internal sense of peace may often be ruffled, eliciting discord or even anger within. Yet harmony-loving Libras are more inclined to repress these "ugly" emotions than outwardly express them. While you are no doubt known for grace under pressure, continually suppressing negative feelings can contribute to a sense of discord and even out-of-character outbursts. Scarlet Monkeyflower can help you honestly connect with and express your full range of feelings so you can maintain emotional poise.

PRETTY FACE (*TRITELEIA IXIOIDES*)

Libras like to look their best, as it helps them feel their best. Yet focusing too much on your physical appearance can be stressful, draining your energy, time, and even cash flow. Pretty Face flower essence can help break the pattern of being overly identified with your external image, helping you see that you are more than just a pretty face and that your true source of beauty lies deep within.

 # Yoga Poses

Yoga can help Libras foster strength and flexibility in their bodies and equanimity in their minds.

TREE (*VRKSASANA*)

Tree, one of the basic balance postures in yoga, can help reinforce a Libra's sense of equilibrium. The key to balancing, as every Libra may know, is to be strong yet supple—just like a tree.

- Stand tall with your feet together. After shifting your weight to your right foot, lift your left leg, externally rotating your thigh in order to rest the sole of your left foot along your inner right thigh or calf. Bring your palms together in front of your heart, lightly gazing at a spot several feet (centimeters) in front of you to help you balance. Eventually spread your arms out to your side—and then toward the ceiling—to help you balance, while imagining them growing like branches. Stay in the posture for up to one minute. Return to the original standing pose, and repeat on the other side.

LORD OF THE DANCE (*NATARAJASANA*)

This elegant asana allows Libras to express their gracefulness. In addition to inspiring balance, this standing posture helps tone the lumbar muscles, lengthen the lower spine, and stimulate the kidneys.

- Stand tall with your feet together. After shifting your weight to your right foot, lift your left leg behind you, bending your knee so that your foot is reaching toward your buttocks. Grab your left foot with your left hand. Push your foot into your hand, which will help you work toward engaging your left hamstring and gluteal muscles as you bring your foot closer to the sky. As you do this, stretch your right arm in front of you or up toward the sky, as you elongate your spine and open your front body into a beautiful backbend. Stay in the pose for up to thirty seconds, and then repeat on the other side.

BOAT (*NAVASANA*)

Boat pose provides an alternative way—a seated posture—in which to practice balance. This posture strengthens the core muscles of the body and may energize the kidneys.

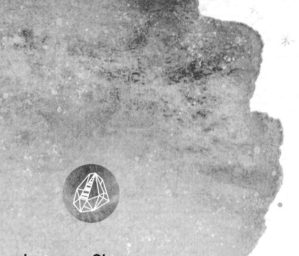

Inspiring Sleep

If you go to bed mad it may keep you from readily getting sleep. This may be especially true if the object of your upset sleeps right beside you. Making the effort to strike a pre-slumber peace accord, whether with your bedmate or a friend with whom you've had a disagreement, may do wonders. It will offer you the harmony necessary to drift off to sleep, giving you the focus and energy you need the next day to work through your relationship tangle.

■ Sit on the floor with your knees bent and your feet on the floor. Hold the back of your lower thighs with your hands. Your sternum should be lifted and your torso slightly leaning back. Rock back so that your feet come off the floor and you're balancing on your sit bones. Have your shins parallel to the floor, or if possible, try to straighten your legs. Remove your hands, straightening your arms so that they point toward your feet and are parallel to the floor. Stay in the pose for one minute.

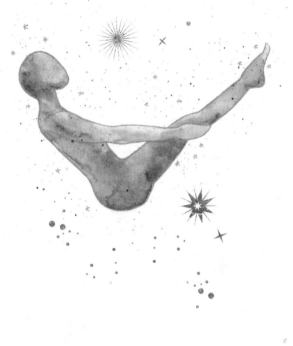

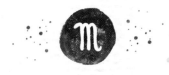

SCORPIO

CHARACTERISTICS

Brooding, complex, determined, emotional, forceful, intense, passionate, probing, regenerative, resilient, resourceful, secretive.

SYMBOL

The Scorpion, an animal known for thriving in the dark, stealthily moving in the shadows, and protecting itself with its venomous sting. In mythological and cultural traditions, the Scorpion is the guardian of the entrance to the underworld and a symbol of protection and retribution.

PLANETARY RULER

Pluto, now considered a dwarf planet. Pluto was the Roman god of the underworld. His counterpart in Greek mythology was Hades. In astrology, Pluto represents power, transformation, and the cycles of life. Mars—embodying desire, courage, and action—is this sign's traditional ruler.

ELEMENT

Water, which embraces the fluid energy of emotion, reflection, and nonlinear understanding. It is sensitive, personal, and responsive. Feelings, empathy, and soulful connections energize water signs while excess rationality, lack of personal space, and inability to access their intuition may deplete their vitality.

MODALITY

Fixed, which adores the planning and building phase of a creative project. Fixed signs prize reliability, predictability, and stamina. Discontinuity or too much change may throw them off their A-game.

Personal Health Profile

Scorpios have incredible regenerative abilities that can serve as powerful allies in their personal health care. You have a cogent capacity to heal yourself, aided by a deep-seated awareness that your mind and emotions play an inextricable role in your physical well-being.

When Scorpios don't feel up to par, they don't just settle into passivity or even self-pity. After all, Scorpios are charter members of the Nietzschean-inspired "what doesn't kill us makes us stronger" club. You'll dive right in with deep resolve to counter any challenges you may face. And since Scorpios are the detectives of the zodiac, you'll passionately commit to finding the cause of and solution to any malady, leaving no stone unturned as you search for answers in places that others may never even consider looking.

When it comes to a wellness routine, Scorpios would much rather work hard, marshalling their formidable inner strength, than be passive or pampered. You like transformative experiences in which you can come up against—and subsequently raze—your perceived limitations, allowing you to plunge more deeply into the substrata of your personal power. Therefore, to rid yourself of impurities and regenerate your body and mind, you're likely to be attracted to the intensity provided by boot camp workouts, detox diets, deep-tissue massages, and other activities that challenge your will and resilience.

Maintaining control and personal power is a central theme in a Scorpio's life. If you feel under the weather, you probably keep it to yourself. You may reason that you don't need others' help, plus you're not inclined to risk having someone perceive you as weak. After all, Scorpios want to be in charge of their destinies and don't want to give any other impression.

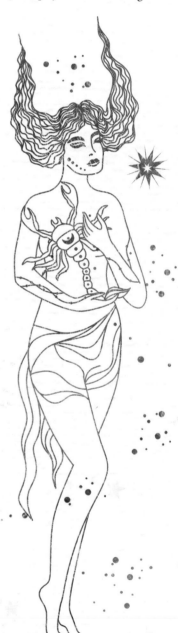

As with all realms, you'll dedicate yourself to doing reams of research to find the most qualified health-care practitioner. Even still, you may put them through the wringer, as you don't necessarily trust people—even a supposed authority—right off the bat. Yet once they prove themselves to be a loyal ally, you'll find yourself deeply committed to their being your partner in health.

Areas of Health Focus

The parts of the body associated with Scorpio include:

- The **large intestine**, which hosts the last stage of digestion and the processing of undigested food for final passage out of the body

- The **urinary tract** and **bladder**, which excrete filtered metabolic waste products

- The **pelvic region**, **genitals**, and **reproductive organs**, which allow you to experience pleasure and create life

Your Scorpionic deep resolve, powerful regenerative capacity, and ability to dig deep to find solutions are some of the resources you can use when facing any health challenge.

CURB HABITS THAT UNDERMINE HEALTH

Scorpios tend to submerge themselves in a sea of feelings. While this stygian journey into your emotional recesses speaks to your sign's inherent need for plumbing the depths, if you don't come up to the surface every now and then, it can leave you feeling overwhelmed. Looking for a way to cope with the intensity, Scorpios often turn to a bottle of wine, a pack of cigarettes, yet another cup of coffee, or some other drug of choice. While going to the dark is part of your nature, take a flashlight with you—in the form of support from friends or family, a therapist, or a detached attitude. That way you are more likely to avoid behaviors that can put your health at risk.

MAINTAIN REGULARITY

While a complex Scorpio might not consider themselves to be "regular," when it comes to your health, being regular is important, especially because your sign rules the large intestine. Bowel irregularity, often experienced as bouts of constipation, can reduce energy, impede weight loss, and detract from a sense of vitality. A fiber-rich diet can help keep things moving smoothly and promote optimal intestinal health. Activities that reduce stress—including exercise, yoga, and meditation—are also beneficial for the resilient Scorpio's digestive health.

PROTECT AGAINST UTIS

While Scorpios may crave intensity, even they don't like the kind of intense symptoms that accompany an infection of the urinary tract, a part of the body ruled by your sign. You can reduce your chances of getting a urinary tract infection (UTI) by doing some simple things: drink lots of water, wear breathable cotton underwear, and empty your bladder before and after having intercourse. If you do get an infection and have to use antibiotics, consider taking probiotics as well. These supplements will help safeguard your beneficial intestinal flora from those antibacterial medications.

EMBRACE ALL STAGES OF LIFE

The transformative ability to create new life—and the reproductive organs with that facility—fall under the domain of Scorpio. Consequently, both menses and menopause are associated with your sign. Female Scorpios are obviously not the only ones to experience these biological events. But, as one whose nature thrives on metamorphosis, a Scorpio may experience these life processes on an exceptionally deep psychological level. While whole foods, natural remedies, and yoga can help smooth out the hormonal roller coaster that both menses and menopause bring, embracing each stage of your womanhood as it unfolds can be deeply healing as well.

 # Healthy Eating Tips

Eating is a transformative Scorpionic experience; after all, the foods you consume get broken down so your body can rebuild and remake itself. That's why nutrient-rich whole foods are so important, as they provide your body with the resources it needs for optimal replenishment.

DON'T RELY ON FOOD FOR SOLACE

Scorpios are passionate creatures. The feelings you experience can seem so deep and all-consuming that you probably imagine that no one, save a fellow Scorpio, can comprehend them. Therefore, if solace can't be found in a relationship, you may seek it elsewhere, which is where emotional eating can come into play. Unfortunately, eating as a refuge from intense emotions doesn't solve any problems—it just creates new ones. Before seeking consolation in a box of cookies, stop and ask yourself what else you can do to feel supported instead. If you find it hard to curb emotional eating, keep carrots, celery, or jicama on hand; munching on them can provide the cathartic release you seek without the caloric baggage.

TRY A DETOX DIET

Like the mythic phoenix, a Scorpio understands that new life can emerge only after the old one is relinquished. Following a detox diet can help you experience this deep regeneration on a physical level, as it allows your body to eliminate compounds that may tax your vitality. And since Scorpios like to challenge their will, and limiting food intake is nothing if not challenging, you're likely to find this process engaging as well. Detox diets can range from a one-day fast to weeks of avoiding all suspected food allergens; tune into your body to find the approach that feels best for you. Take note, though: with a tendency to go to extremes, Scorpios need to view a detox diet as a periodic healing ritual rather than an ongoing dietary approach.

PRACTICE MODERATION

Scorpios have a tendency to go to extremes. Whatever you do, you commit to and do with full force, diving deep into the experience, which provides you with the emotional charge you crave. Yet if you go to extremes with your eating habits—for example, bingeing and/or being overly restrictive with your food intake—it can have less-than-supportive effects on your health. Not only can extreme eating behaviors lead to unhealthy weight gain or loss, but they can also affect your nerves, metabolism, and mental outlook. Exploring your relationship with food under the guidance of a skilled nutritionist may provide you with deep insights into yourself, something that Scorpios crave.

 # Health-Supporting Foods

Scorpios may have an affinity to foods that are deeply colored and intense in flavor. Foods to which you may be drawn include dark chocolate, fermented foods, cranberries, and beverages.

DARK CHOCOLATE

Scorpios' love of the dark can come in handy when choosing chocolate with the most health benefits. Darker chocolates have a higher content of cacao and therefore a greater amount of heart-healthy flavonoid antioxidants. Chocolate's allure also extends to its reputation as an aphrodisiac, a boon for passionate Scorpios. Some ideas to add chocolate to recipes include grating some on top of a fresh berry salad and mixing cocoa powder and honey into plain yogurt for a healthy dessert. While chocolate may have benefits, it's not, unfortunately, a cure-all. So curb the Scorpionic tendency to overindulge, and instead enjoy this treat in moderation.

FERMENTED FOODS

Scorpios are masters of change; as you transform and evolve, you become more connected to your inherent power. The same can be said for fermented foods and beverages. For example, when bacterial cultures are added to milk, the result is foods that are easier to digest, such as yogurt and kefir. Additionally, the beneficial bacteria added to ferment foods can help repopulate your own supply of health-giving intestinal flora. Look for high-quality yogurts that include an array of live active bacterial cultures. Kefir is a delicious drinkable alternative to yogurt. Sauerkraut and kimchi, the spicy Korean side dish, are flavorful accompaniments to a variety of dishes. The popular beverage kombucha is created through fermenting sugar-sweetened tea, while its cousin, jun, is made from tea and honey.

CRANBERRIES

Cranberries, like Scorpios, are known for their sharp bite and powerful healing abilities. While strongly associated with Thanksgiving fare, cranberries now commonly appear in dishes throughout the year. Their growing popularity is related to research that shows this little antioxidant-rich fruit to be a potent weapon against developing infections of the Scorpio-ruled urinary tract. To avoid empty calories, purchase cranberry juice concentrate—which you can reconstitute with water and a little natural sweetener—instead of presweetened cranberry juice cocktail. It's easy to make your own cranberry sauce: just simmer fresh or frozen berries in honey-sweetened orange juice for about fifteen minutes, until they split or pop open.

Wellness Therapies

If you set your mind on transformation, you'll do whatever is necessary—including partaking in a host of wellness therapies—to achieve it.

STRUCTURAL INTEGRATION

A powerful form of bodywork, Structural Integration targets the soft tissue web known as fascia, the covering that envelops muscles, nerves, and bones. Releasing tight fascia is thought to transform deep-seated patterns of misalignment, leading to reduced chronic pain and freer motion. Rolfing and Soma are two popular methods of Structural Integration. Like a Scorpio, this bodywork therapy goes deep, so you may experience slight discomfort during a session; however, if any zodiac sign is able to handle a bit of temporary pain for long-lasting gain, it's a Scorpio. Structural Integration treatments are often organized into ten sessions, and therefore requires a commitment; yet as Scorpios are nothing if not committed, this may not be a challenge for you.

COLONICS

As a Scorpio, you don't shy away from things, even those that other people find unseemly and crude, if you believe that there is some merit in experiencing them. Therefore, not only may you be intrigued by the idea of a colonic but also really appreciate the benefits that this treatment can offer. By infusing water into the Scorpio-ruled large intestine, colonics help flush out excess waste materials from the body. Proponents note that this aids in both detoxification and better digestion. Just make sure to find a colon hydrotherapist who is licensed and uses sterile disposable equipment. Ask the therapist to recommend foods or supplements that can replenish any good intestinal bacteria that may get washed away during a treatment.

FLOATATION TANKS

Floatation tanks feature three things Scorpios love: water, darkness, and time to connect with your feelings. While Scorpios have an affinity for plunging below, in these tanks your body hovers on the surface, thanks to the water's very high salt concentration. Floatation tanks may lead to buoyant health; research studies suggest that they have beneficial effects for those with sleep difficulties, anxiety, and muscle tension. If you can't make it to a float center, you can do a modified version at home. Make your bathroom as dark as possible, use a pink noise machine to tamp down ambient sounds, and don an eye mask while bathing. And while you may not be able to add enough Epsom salts to achieve the level of buoyancy you experience in a float tank, you can still enjoy a tranquility-inspiring experience.

Relaxation Practices

Scorpios can relax the most when they feel safe expressing their uniquely deep natures, which like to discover hidden truths.

NEO-TANTRA

Scorpios have an affinity for provocative experiences that allow them to transcend their egos, enabling their deeper selves to emerge. As such, you may gain great benefit from practicing neo-tantra, a modern-day translation of the Buddhist and Hindu disciplines that honor sex as a vehicle for spiritual elevation. Neo-tantric rituals focus on stimulating the body's energy centers (known as chakras), honoring the deep essence of your partner, and experiencing sex as a consciousness-elevating experience. While there are many books available on the subject, taking a workshop is also an option. Given these courses offer varying degrees of exploration, thoroughly research the teacher and how the course is organized before signing up.

MYSTERIES

Adept at clueing into others' hidden motives and equipped with a keen interest in leaving no stone unturned, a Scorpio loves a good mystery. Indulging your inner sleuth by burying yourself in a detective novel or bingeing a suspense-filled miniseries is a great way for a Scorpio to unwind. If you want a more lifelike whodunit experience, consider attending a mystery theater performance. You can also start a book club focused on mystery fiction or true crime novels, or buy a whodunit game kit and invite some friends over for a deadly good time. And, if you'd rather listen than read, survey the scores of podcasts focused on this genre.

MUD TREATMENT

Scorpios like exploring a full range of experiences and don't mind getting their hands a little dirty, both figuratively and literally, in the process. So why not get your whole body dirty to clean up your health by enjoying a mud treatment? Being mired in mineral-rich mud, whether as a body or facial mask, can help relax your muscles, as well as improve circulation and aid in detoxification. You can purchase mud masks in pharmacies and stores that sell beauty products. Also, similar to mud, ventilated green clay can be used at home for healing poultices that can help relieve joint and muscle pain. Mud treatments are also known as fangotherapy or pelotherapy.

 # Natural Remedies

When it comes to your health-care practitioners, watch for your tendency to be secretive: tell them which natural remedies you use to be assured that none will negatively interact with medications you may take.

ALOE VERA (*ALOE VERA*)

Scorpio is a sign of timeless endurance; similarly, aloe vera was traditionally viewed as a symbol of eternal life. Aloe's regenerative properties provide great benefits when applied topically, helping to soften skin, heal cuts, and temper burns. Aloe vera juice is also one of the premier natural laxatives, a helpful remedy when the Scorpio-ruled intestine needs a little extra support. Look for juice products that contain at least 99 percent aloe vera. For back-to-the-earth healing, buy an aloe plant; set it on a sunny sill, breaking open a leaf and extracting the gel when your skin needs some soothing.

FLAXSEED (*LINUM USITATISSIMUM*)

Flaxseed is an incredibly rich source of fiber, helping to promote the health of the Scorpio-ruled large intestine as well as lower cholesterol. With its rich concentration of lignin phytonutrients, a type of insoluble fiber, it is acclaimed for balancing hormone levels and reducing breast cancer risk in postmenopausal women. Additionally, flaxseed contains a large concentration of anti-inflammatory omega-3 fatty acids. While flaxseed is thought of as a supplement, it can also be enjoyed as a food incorporated into your daily diet. For better absorption—and therefore greater benefits—it's important to use ground, rather than whole, flaxseed.

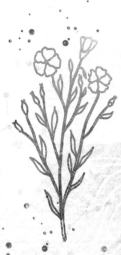

BLACK COHOSH (*ACTAEA RACEMOSA*)

Black cohosh may be of benefit for Scorpios with painful periods or premenstrual syndrome. In several studies, it has also been found to provide relief from menopausal symptoms, such as hot flashes, insomnia, and anxiety. These female health benefits are not just recent discoveries, however. For centuries, Native Americans have used it for a variety of gynecological challenges. As black cohosh may have mild estrogen-like activity, if you take estrogenic medications or have concern about your estrogen levels, consult a physician before using this herb. Black cohosh preparations are made from the rhizome and root parts of the plant.

 ## Essential Oils

Aromatherapy is a deeply alchemical process, something that transformation-inclined Scorpios will appreciate.

YLANG-YLANG (*CANANGA ODORATA*)

Sex can be a very powerful experience for a Scorpio. Yet, if you deny your innate sensual nature, libidinal lethargy can set in. If your hots are a little cool, try ylang-ylang, one of the most well-known aphrodisiac scents. You needn't scatter ylang-ylang flowers on your bed as some newly married couples in Indonesia do—just add the flower's essential oil to your personal care repertoire. Ylang-ylang makes a sultry perfume. For a twist on the traditional Indonesian marriage bed, you can spritz your linens with a mixture of ylang-ylang and water. Or, add a few drops of ylang-ylang to coconut oil, and apply as a South Pacific–inspired hair treatment.

BASIL (*OCIMUM BASILICUM*)

According to superstition, basil leaves could transform themselves into your astrological totem, the Scorpion. While this may be folkloric fancy, basil essential oil can certainly transform your health. It is said to integrate the conscious and unconscious minds, promoting psychic vision. It is also suggested to have anti-inflammatory properties. Basil essential oil also is thought to reduce menstruation-associated pain (yet, owing to its stimulating properties, it's best to avoid it during pregnancy). Inhale this fragrance when you want to relax and feel centered. And, as it can also act as an insect repellent, applying body lotion with a few drops of basil essential oil may help keep vexing critters away.

HELICHRYSUM (*HELICHRYSUM ITALICUM*)

Like your sign, helichrysum—also known as everlasting—is prized for its regenerative abilities. As such, it is thought to be one of the best oils to use for healing scars and wounds. When it comes to healing emotional scarring and wounds, the scent of helichrysum is also well suited. It helps unblock deep subconscious emotions and stimulates a profound level of self-compassion, something with which a Scorpio may need assistance at times. To help untangle knotted emotional energy, use helichrysum in a room diffuser to enjoy an uplifting environment. Add a few drops to massage oil for relief of aches and pain, or to some moisturizer to bolster skin health.

 ## Flower Essences

Flower essences evoke deep changes in one's psychological and emotional well-being, great for Scorpios looking for ways to be more aligned with their truly powerful natures. (See page 20 for how to use flower essences.)

HOLLY (*ILEX AQUIFOLIUM*)

Suspicious Scorpios don't often share the full range of their feelings with others (after all, you may reason, "Who would understand?"). Accordingly, you may believe that others aren't as candid with you either. If your distrust paves the way toward isolation and anger, Holly flower essence may be a great remedy for you. It can help open your heart to the possibility that even if others have feelings and motives that they don't share with you, their intentions may still come from a benevolent place. Additionally, it can also help remedy a feeling of separateness in which Scorpios sometimes swim, inspiring a reminder that everyone is truly connected.

MUSTARD (*SINAPIS ARVENSIS*)

Scorpios seem to have a closer relationship with the subconscious than many others. While this gives you the ability to experience an expansive range of powerful feelings, it can also engender a sense of gloom that seems to come out of nowhere. Understanding the reasons for your feelings can deepen your self-awareness and also reduce the potential for being blindsided by seemingly out-of-the-blue mood swings. This is the realm of Mustard flower essence, which can help you plumb the emotional heaviness and further shed light on the cause of the darkness that may reside within.

BASIL (*OCIMUM BASILICUM*)

As the Scorpionic nature has a great affinity for the powerful and the intense, sex can be a potent avenue for experiencing profound emotions and interpersonal connection. It can also help you get in touch with your deep creative energies. However, if you feel shame concerning your sexuality (whether from past trauma or societal pressures), you may employ sensuality in ways that are not truly aligned with your emotions and desires. If you feel that your sex life is polarized from your heart's intentions, try Basil flower essence, which can help you reclaim and reintegrate this dynamic and joyfully creative part of yourself.

 Yoga Poses

With Scorpio being a fixed sign, the practice of yoga is beneficial for you because it can inspire flexibility in both body and mind.

GARLAND (*MALASANA*)

Intense like a Scorpio, this wide squat pose is sure to unfasten any tightness in your pelvis, stretching your groin and bringing energy to your genital region. It also benefits the urinary tract, and, as you'll notice, is an amazing hip opener.

■ With your feet close together, move into a squat, separating your knees so they are slightly wider than your torso. (If you can't keep your heels on the floor, place a rolled-up blanket underneath them.) Reach your torso forward with your arms outstretched. Then swing your arms around the outside of your legs, reaching for the backs of your ankles with your hands. Hold this position for up to one minute.

WIDE-ANGLE SEATED FORWARD BEND (*UPAVISTHA KONASANA*)

While Scorpios aren't known for compromise, you may like this seemingly compromising position, as it can be a great teacher. It allows you to see how you respond when you meet your limits, fostering an ability to accept your boundaries with emotional honesty.

- Sit on the floor, or a folded blanket, with your legs straight in front of you and your spine elongated. Open your legs out to the sides as far as feels comfortable. Ground your legs, making sure both your knees and toes are pointing upward. With a lengthened torso, tip your pelvis toward the ground, leaning forward. Place your hands on the ground, finding a position that stretches your inner legs and hamstrings. Stay in the pose for up to two minutes.

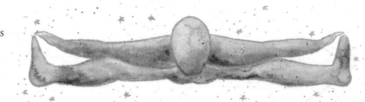

DEAD BUG (*ANANDA BALASANA*)

It takes a special breed—notably a Scorpio who is fascinated by the darker things in life—to appreciate a posture called Dead Bug. This asana is at once gently restorative (allowing you to maintain a sense of control) and intensely provocative (as your groin and leg muscles succumb to a state of relaxation).

- Lie on your back with your knees bent and your feet touching the floor. Slowly raise your legs and tip them toward your torso, grabbing the outsides of your feet. Ideally, your feet should be above your knees with your shins perpendicular to the floor. Gently

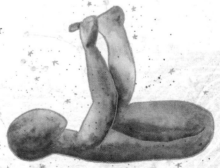

pull your feet toward your hips so that your knees come closer to the sides of your torso. Keep your lower back lengthened and pressed down toward the ground. Stay in the pose for up to one minute.

Inspiring Sleep

Do you know one of the things that Scorpios and good sleep hygiene have in common? The love of the dark. That's because melatonin, the slumber-inspiring hormone, is released in darkness, and if not enough is produced it can disturb our sleep cycles. If light streams in the room, get blackout curtains or wear an eye mask to safeguard your journey to the land of Nod. Eliminate or reduce other sources of light as well; avoid clocks with bright, digital readouts and turn your phone to airplane mode when you sleep so that notifications do not illuminate the room and disturb your slumber.

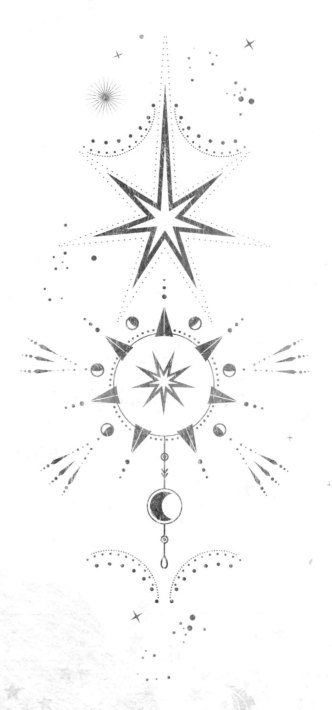

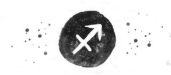

SAGITTARIUS

CHARACTERISTICS

Adventurous, dogmatic, exuberant, inspired, jovial, optimistic, philosophical, upbeat, versatile, visionary, wise, zealous.

SYMBOL

The Archer, pictured as a centaur, a mythic half-horse/half-human creature that represents the melding of our animal and spiritual natures. In mythological and cultural traditions, the centaur is a symbol of adventure, revelry, wisdom, and courage.

PLANETARY RULER

Jupiter, the largest planet in our solar system. Jupiter was the Roman king of the gods, who governed the universe. His counterpart in Greek mythology was Zeus. In astrology, Jupiter represents understanding, growth, good fortune, and faith.

ELEMENT

Fire, characterized by the dynamic energy of inspiration, enthusiasm, and passion. It is transformative, kinetic, and action oriented. Movement, spontaneity, and tapping into their imagination energizes fire signs while slowness, stagnancy, and a sense of limitation may deplete their vitality.

MODALITY

Mutable, which has an affinity for the adjustment and finessing stage of a creative project. Mutable signs are flexible, adaptive, and chameleon-like. They may find themselves agitated if things are too structured or overly defined.

Personal Health Profile

As with everything in their lives, Sagittarius are apt to take a philosophical approach to their health. You seek the deeper meaning in all things. With *why* as one of your favorite words, you may question, for example, *why* you may experience certain health challenges or *why* one wellness approach works more effectively for you than another. This inquiring nature that pursues insightful answers is elemental to Sagittarus's ability to live a full and healthful life.

Rather than relying solely on health-care practitioners for wellness wisdom, Sagittarius seeks it from a large sphere of resources. From friends to coworkers, health books to spiritual texts, the Archer aims to find a framework that will allow them access to truth and significance, the Sagittarian Holy Grail.

While a Sagittarius's spirited approach to living brings much pleasure, it may also pose health challenges. For example, being so enthusiastic, you may have a hard time acknowledging your limits. This can result in exhaustion or even reckless injuries, both avoidable by taking a slower, more deliberate approach to the task at hand.

Sagittarius loves to celebrate any occasion—including just the adventure of another day— and these festivities often involve food and drink. If not enjoyed in moderation (a concept that doesn't come easily to the Archer), you may be prone to weight issues, especially later in life. Additionally, drinking alcohol and consuming fatty foods may pose extra challenges to your liver, an organ associated with your sign.

While your abundant energy and fiery constitution normally provide you with a strong sense of health, when you do fall ill, take comfort in the fact that you have amazing healing resources at hand. In addition to the deep level of understanding you seek, you always set your sights high and pursue your goals with gusto. If optimal well-being is your aim, as a Sagittarius, you'll travel far and wide to find the ways to achieve it. When combined with your profound level of faith, you hold an almost magical recipe for overcoming many wellness obstacles.

Areas of Health Focus

The parts of the body associated with Sagittarius include:

- The **liver**, the body's largest organ, responsible for detoxifying chemicals, producing fat-digesting bile, and numerous other vital functions
- The **thighs** and **buttocks**, both necessary for journeying and locomotion
- The **hips**, **sacrum**, and **coccyx**, which provide you with stability and movement
- The **sciatic nerve**, the longest and widest nerve, which runs from the lower back all the way to the feet

Your Sagittarian spirited energy, deep well of faith, and motivation to learn new things are some of the resources you can use when facing any health challenge.

LOVE YOUR LIVER

Just like the god Jupiter, the Sagittarius-ruled liver performs numerous functions to maintain order, all in the name of supporting well-being. These include the filtration of blood, the detoxification of chemicals, the production of fat-metabolizing bile, and the storage of glycogen (a source of energy). One important way to support hepatic health is to reduce the burden placed on the liver's detoxification systems. To do so, watch your intake of alcohol and synthetic food additives, and choose organic over conventionally grown produce whenever you can. Also to this end, reduce your reliance on synthetically based household cleaners, opting for their more natural counterparts instead.

STRENGTHEN YOUR MUSCLES

The sign of Sagittarius represents the desire to move from place to place, exploring the world and learning all that it has to teach. Consequently, it makes sense that the buttocks and thighs, two related areas intimately connected to movement, are associated with your sign. If the muscles located in these areas—notably the quadriceps, hamstrings, or gluteus muscles—are overly tight or weak, it can lead to lower back pain, knee instability, or sciatic nerve impingement. Regular exercise and massage can keep your muscles toned. Also, if you have a desk job, honor your Sagittarian need to move, and walk around every hour or so to rev up the blood flow to your lower body.

STABILIZE HIP HEALTH

Symbols of female sexuality as well as fertility, the hips are another Sagittarius-ruled area of the body central to locomotion. An assortment of conditions—including arthritis, osteoporosis, and hamstring strains—can affect the hips' range of motion and cause pain. Exercise approaches that strengthen and stabilize the hip socket and surrounding muscles can be beneficial; these include Pilates (see page 139), with its focus on muscle lengthening, and Gyrotonics, which targets joint mobilization. Additionally, making sure your diet is rich in bone-building nutrients—such as calcium, magnesium, vitamin D, and vitamin K—can help prevent osteoporosis in the hips.

AVOID SPORTS INJURIES

Engaging in sports and fitness is a great outlet for an Archer's abundant physical energy and competitive nature. Yet it's also an arena in which you need to take extra care. Enthusiastic Sagittarius are known to push themselves beyond their limits (*limits, what limits?* is a common Sagittarian refrain). This can put you at risk for strains, sprains, and other sports-related injuries. Don't forget to warm up and cool down before and after exercise, which is especially important as you age. Also, keep yourself well hydrated and nourished. These tips will help transform your athletic pursuits into feats of glory rather than bouts of injury.

Healthy Eating Tips

Enjoying food and drink is one means by which Sagittarius enthusiastically participates in the joyful adventure called life. Yet with great exuberance may come a tendency toward overindulgence, something on which the Archer should keep tabs.

ENJOY LIVER-SUPPORTING FOODS

Foods that maintain liver health include those rich in sulfur, such as onions, garlic, and the brassica vegetables (for example, cauliflower, kale, and broccoli). Onions go great in just about anything from soups to salads, meat-centered entrées to vegetarian stir-fries. Garlic and lemon, mixed with a touch of extra virgin olive oil, is a delicious liver-supporting dressing to top lightly steamed brassica vegetables. For optimal hepatic health, you'll also want to limit your consumption of alcohol; be festive instead by enjoying a delicious non-alcoholic mocktail beverage. Also, curb your consumption of high-fat foods, synthetic additives, and foods grown with pesticides, since the liver has to work overtime to break down these compounds.

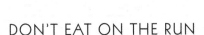

DON'T EAT ON THE RUN

With so many paths to pursue and adventures to experience, a Sagittarius's schedule is brimming with appointments, social engagements, and activities. As such, the Archer often noshes while on the go, which can create challenges to eating healthfully. By not planning out meals, nourishment can often mean grabbing what's convenient and on hand, which is more than likely something that's packaged, processed, and laden with carbs. Take the time to pack snacks when you know you will be on the run all day. This will help you tide over your appetite and not give in to impulsive food choices. Some ideas include cut-up broccoli, baby carrots, trail mix, bananas, and organic energy bars.

EXPLORE CULINARY GLOBE-TROTTING

Sagittarius are the travelers of the zodiac. Even if you aren't able to traverse the world physically, one way to experience the glories of the globe is to sample the unique food offerings of different cultures. By exploring international cuisines—whether by eating at ethnic restaurants or learning to cook these foods yourself—you'll expand your horizons and learn new things, a raison d'être of any Sagittarius. Embark on your culinary trek by visiting a bookstore and exploring its selection of world-cuisine recipe books. Take a cooking class at a local community college, adult learning center, or natural foods market, and learn how to make tapas, mix curry blends, or prepare dim sum.

 ## Health-Supporting Foods

Many healthy foods—including olives and hazelnuts—are associated with your sign. Appreciative of other cultures' wisdom, Sagittarius would do well to incorporate the South American grains quinoa and amaranth into their diets.

OLIVES AND OLIVE OIL

Sports-loving Sagittarius may be interested to know that olive wreaths and olive oil were some of the prizes awarded to ancient Olympic athletes. Today, Jupiter-ruled olives and their oil still earn a gold medal when it comes to nutrition. Rich in health-promoting fats and antioxidants, olives and olive oil play a starring role in the Mediterranean diet and are thought to be one of the reasons that this approach to eating offers protection against cardiovascular disease and cancer. Sampling different varieties of olives—Kalamata, Picholine, Cerignola, and Castelvetrano, to name just a few—can be a delicious adventure. Opt for extra virgin olive oil—rather than virgin or refined—as it has the highest concentration of antioxidants.

HAZELNUTS

If wisdom comes with age, then Jupiter-ruled hazelnuts are a very intelligent food. Ancient Greek physicians praised the curative properties of hazelnuts. And even further back in time, close to five thousand years ago, the Chinese considered hazelnuts to be a very sacred food. Their track record for health-giving properties continues to this day, as they are a very rich source of many nutrients, including magnesium, manganese, vitamin E, and monounsaturated fat. Enjoy hazelnuts by tossing them onto salads or adding them to trail mix. For a Spanish twist on a pesto recipe, substitute hazelnuts and Manchego cheese for pine nuts and Parmesan. Hazelnut oil has a high smoke point, making it a great choice for sautés and stir-fries.

QUINOA AND AMARANTH

If you're a Sagittarius looking for a sustained energy boost—whether for exercise or just life's daily adventures—try quinoa and amaranth. These ancient foods—revered by the Incan, Mayan, and Aztec cultures—are rich in complex carbohydrates and fiber. Enjoyed like whole grains, gluten-free quinoa and amaranth are actually seeds that feature a well-rounded supply of all the essential amino acids, making them a good source of protein. Before cooking quinoa, wash it well to remove its saponin compound, which can impart a soapy taste to this otherwise delicious food. Amaranth has a porridge-like texture, so you may want to cook it with brown rice if you'd like to enjoy a dish with a more grain-like consistency.

 # Wellness Therapies

Wellness therapies can be an active and engaging way to further your pursuit of well-being.

THAI MASSAGE

If you seek a style of bodywork that's suited to your spirited temperament and appreciation for the wisdom of other cultures, try Thai massage. During a Thai massage session, you rest fully clothed on a padded floor mat while the practitioner stretches your muscles and mobilizes your joints by moving you into various yogalike postures. They then apply pressure—with their hands, feet, elbows, or knees—to release tension in your muscles and connective tissue. In Thailand and other Asian countries, this form of bodywork is often called *nuat phaen boran*. This translates into "ancient-style massage," a term you may see used to describe this form of healing art.

PILATES

The enhanced strength and postural alignment that come from doing Pilates will help the Archer hold steady aim at any target on the horizon. During a Pilates session, you work with a trained instructor on a series of movement exercises, either on specialized machines or floor mats. In addition to core-strengthening benefits, Pilates fosters greater body awareness and muscle control as well as healthier breathing habits. Before you commit to a particular Pilates instructor, compare the background and experience of several to see which one aligns best with you. Many gyms and studios offer group Pilates-style mat classes, which you can take in person or online.

EQUINE-ASSISTED PSYCHOTHERAPY

If, in your quest to better understand yourself, you've been considering psychotherapy, you may be interested in exploring equine-assisted psychotherapy (EAP). Led by a trained mental health counselor and featuring horses to facilitate therapeutic benefit, EAP is especially well suited to Sagittarius, as your sign is symbolized by the mythic centaur. Through interacting with the horse, you can build self-confidence and learn new relationship skills. In addition to EAP, there are other therapies that feature horses as vehicles for enhancing well-being. For example, hippotherapy focuses on improving coordination, balance, and functional movement skills rather than on psychotherapeutic healing.

 # Relaxation Practices

As Archers are so adept at using their minds, imaginations, and active spirits to attract that which they seek, engaging in relaxation practices may be an enjoyable and fruitful quest.

CREATIVE VISUALIZATION

Sagittarius has an uncanny ability to manifest good fortune; it is as if your positive attitude, expansive vision, and unequivocal faith constitute a secret recipe for attracting treasured outcomes. With this ability, you would be a natural at creative visualization, a stress-relieving technique that engages your conscious and subconscious minds to work in unison to help you meet your chosen goals. There are numerous written and audio books available to help you learn creative visualization techniques. Not only can this relaxation practice inspire calm, but you can also use it to achieve other goals, such as enhancing athletic performance or reducing muscular tension.

SPORTS-TRAINING PROGRAMS

Being active is often more relaxing to a Sagittarius than sitting still, which is great because exercise is one of the best ways to reduce stress. Yet destination-oriented Sagittarius need a mission, and so exercising for its own sake may be unlikely to sustain your interest. To get fit while honoring your purposeful nature, pick a goal—whether it be completing a 5K walkathon, reducing your golf handicap, or getting in shape for ski season—and focus your fitness routine with this aim in mind. As always, honor your Sagittarian exuberance yet, as you train, be realistic about what you are capable of doing at any one time; this way you can be active while also avoiding exercise-related injuries caused by overexertion.

TRAVEL

Let your arrow fly and follow it on a journey around the world. Exploring foreign countries—connecting with different landscapes and the people who call them home—can be a very enriching experience for a Sagittarius. The message board of travel websites can be great resources for information on hotels, restaurants, and tourist destinations. However, if budgetary or other lifestyle realities keep you from globe-trotting, you can still experience some of its benefits by reading travel memoirs and guidebooks, or exploring travel-oriented television shows or films. Television stations abound with inspiring shows on adventure travel, culinary expeditions, and sightseeing trips around the world.

 # Natural Remedies

The quest of a Sagittarius is that of discovery. Sorting through the multitude of available natural remedies to determine the ones that are best for you can be a very health-rewarding journey.

MILK THISTLE (*SILYBUM MARIANUM*)

An herb dating back to ancient Greco-Roman times, milk thistle is currently one of the most commonly used remedies for liver health. Its popularity stems from its efficacy at providing the Sagittarius-ruled liver with a wide range of benefits, including protecting the liver from exposure to harmful toxins. Milk thistle is also a powerful antioxidant that shields the liver from free radical damage. Milk thistle is commonly available in capsule and tincture form. As many of its benefits have been attributed to its silymarin flavonoids, look for milk thistle remedies standardized to 70 to 80 percent of these compounds.

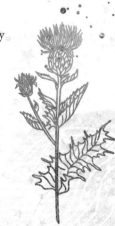

AMLA (*EMBLICA OFFICINALIS*)

If your quest to discover leads you to amla, you're in luck. One of the prized rejuvenating herbs in India and its Ayurvedic medical tradition, amla is said to promote longevity, and is referred to as the "sustainer" in traditional Hindu texts. Not only does amla contain more vitamin C than oranges, but it is also used in Ayurvedic medicine as a liver tonic, a digestive strengthener, an immune system fortifier, and a hair conditioner. Amla is available in either capsule or powder form. You may also find dried amla fruit or pickled preserves in stores that sell Indian food.

CHOLINE

Choline—a B vitamin found in soy foods, egg yolks, and lentils—is a nutrient that offers benefits to the liver as well as other aspects of health. Dietary choline deficiency may lead to fat accumulation in the liver, which can cause inflammation and cell damage if severe. In addition, as a key component of neurons as well as the nervous system messenger acetylcholine, it plays a role in brain health. Choline is available in a variety of forms, including phosphatidylcholine, lecithin, and choline salt (such as choline chloride or bitartrate). Taking choline supplements with meals enhances its absorption.

142

 Essential Oils

That aromatherapy is a healing tradition used by cultures worldwide and features the essential oils of plants from around the globe should make it attractive to internationally interested Sagittarius.

JUNIPER (*JUNIPERUS COMMUNIS*)

Juniper essential oil has far-reaching health benefits for a Sagittarius; it may relieve both muscle cramps and the uncomfortable feeling that comes from overindulging in food and drink. Throughout history, it has also been used in a number of wellness applications; for example, in ancient Greece, juniper was recognized by noted physicians as a powerful liver tonic while also being used by Olympic athletes to enhance endurance. To make an after-exercise muscle-relieving salve, add some juniper to massage oil. To give your energy levels a boost after a night of Sagittarian regaling, use juniper oil in a room diffuser, and revel in its uplifting and detoxifying properties.

GRAPEFRUIT (*CITRUS PARADISI*)

The essential oil of grapefruit is paradise for an Archer on a wellness quest. It helps relieve muscle tension and is a good remedy for quelling joint pain. Grapefruit oil is also said to release stagnant liver *chi* (life force energy), which, according to traditional Chinese medicine, contributes to irritability as well as PMS. Additionally, it helps with fluid retention and may even reduce the cellulite that can appear on the Sagittarius-ruled thighs and buttocks. Apply massage cream scented with grapefruit oil to your hips and thighs if they are beset with aches and pains. A belly balm of grapefruit essence mixed with coconut oil may help with bloating and liver detoxification.

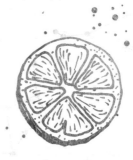

NUTMEG (*MYRISTICA FRAGRANS*)

Nutmeg has long been a symbol of the Sagittarian attribute of good fortune. And, as luck would have it, nutmeg has some great health benefits. Nutmeg is said to allay muscle aches, inspire the mind, and enhance the vividness of dreams. According to medical folklore, people carried nutmeg in their pockets to relieve lower back pain. Carry a vial of nutmeg oil in your bag or briefcase. Not only will this twist on the folkloric tradition provide you with a talisman, but it will also make it easily accessible for times when your mind needs a bit of uplift and expansion. Use nutmeg oil judiciously because large doses may cause side effects.

 # Flower Essences

Wisdom-seeking Sagittarius may appreciate flower essences for their ability to teach you more about yourself, since they can help you understand and overcome some of the stress you may experience. (See page 20 for how to use flower essences.)

VERVAIN (*VERBENA OFFICINALIS*)

Archers are passionate, especially around their ideals and the pursuit of their aspirations. Moderation is not your modus operandi; you're usually all in with your enthusiasm, whether by pushing yourself to great accomplishments or in your energetic appeals to others to adopt the viewpoints you share with them. While you may accomplish great feats, sometimes your overstriving may put you on a pathway to physical exhaustion and nervous tension. When you need to balance your arduous pursuits with some pragmatism and moderation, try Vervain flower essence.

RABBITBRUSH (*ERICAMERIA NAUSEOSA*)

A Sagittarius rarely misses the forest for the trees; rather, the opposite sometimes proves challenging. With your focus on the big picture, you may at times miss the smaller details, thus forgoing additional opportunities for learning. When surveying life, and all the wisdom it yields, if you need assistance being open to nuances that can help you access a wider perspective of understanding, try Rabbitbrush flower essence.

ANGELICA (*ANGELICA ARCHANGELICA*)

Archers are known for their deep faith, their trust that everything has meaning and import, and their belief that every situation eventually works itself out for the greater good. Even so, your faith may be challenged for periods of time, notably during a crisis or important life transition. For guidance during these times, and assistance in restoring your belief in an ordered benevolence, try Angelica flower essence.

 # Yoga Poses

The Archer loves to learn, and yoga can provide you with an unending experience of discovering new postures, spiritual insights, and ways of being mindful in your practice.

WARRIOR II (*VIRABHA-DRASANA II*)

Within the expansively open posture that characterizes Warrior II, you can see the speculative nature of the Archer. In this posture, you gaze into the distance over your outstretched arm, peacefully visualizing a goal that lies ahead just over the horizon.

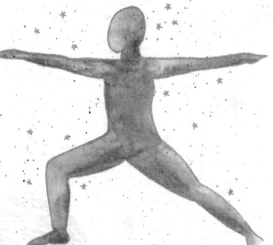

■ Stand tall with your head aligned over the center of your pelvis, your arms outstretched and parallel to the floor, and your palms facing down. Walk your feet about 4 feet (122 cm) apart, rotating your right foot out 90 degrees and your left one in about 30 degrees. Ensure that you feel both stability and ease in your stance. Bend your right knee so it is above your right foot, and point your kneecap toward your middle toe. Extend your arms wide, stretching your shoulder blades while at the same time gazing over the top of your right fingertips. Stay in the pose for up to one minute, and then repeat on the other side.

FIRE LOG (*AGNISTAMBHASANA*)

With the hips as an area of focus for fiery Sagittarius, the intense, hip-opening Fire Log pose can be very beneficial for the Archer. This posture stretches the hip flexors as well as the gluteus and piriformis muscles.

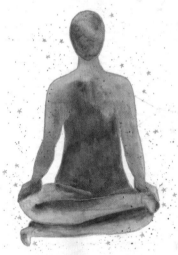

■ Sit on your mat with your knees bent in front of you and the soles of your feet on the ground. Outwardly rotate your right hip so the outside of your right leg falls toward the floor. Adjust your right leg so your shin is parallel to the front of your mat. Place your left ankle on your right knee, with your left shin stacked above your right. If your left knee doesn't reach your right foot, place padding below it for support. Flex your feet and sit up straight. Stay in the pose for up to two minutes, and then switch leg positions.

HIGH LUNGE (*UTTHITA ASHWA SANCHALANASANA*)

High Lunge pose lengthens the Sagittarius-ruled quadricep and psoas muscles. It also teaches an important pearl of yogic wisdom: no matter how many times you do a pose, even one as basic as this, you can always learn new things about your body and breath.

■ Stand tall with your feet together, placing your hands on your hips. Bend forward at your hip joints, bring your palms to the floor (or yoga blocks) in front of your feet, and gently bend your knees. Step your right foot toward the back edge of the mat,

Inspiring Sleep

Sagittarius often prize daytime over sleep time, because they perceive that it's only then that they can have the adventures of which they are so fond. Yet, in addition to being elemental to physical strength and well-being, sleep connects you to a dynamic landscape offering all sorts of exploration— that of your dreams. Working with your dreams can help you tap into a deeper level of self-understanding, which is something you cherish.

positioning your heel so it is above the ball of your foot. Bend your left knee so that it aligns over your ankle. Your hands (or fingertips) should be on the ground on either side of your left foot and your torso should be straight while you lean on your left thigh. Straighten your right leg by pushing strongly through your foot. Try to keep your hips even by pressing into the ground with both of your feet. Stay in the pose for up to one minute, and then repeat on the other side.

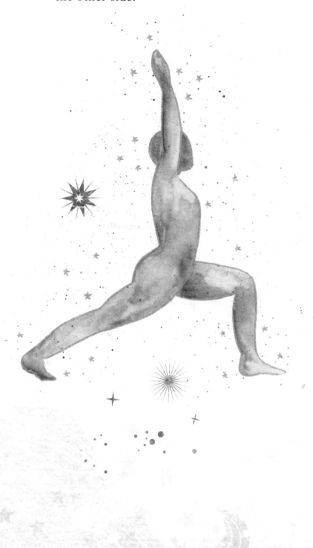

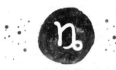

CAPRICORN

CHARACTERISTICS

Ambitious, committed, conservative, disciplined, frugal, hardworking, loyal, persistent, pragmatic, sarcastic, straightforward, structured.

SYMBOL

The Goat, an animal known for its perseverance, sure-footedness, and dedicated guardianship of its resources. It's often represented as a Sea Goat. In mythological and cultural traditions, the Goat is a symbol of prosperity, fertility, and the beneficial elements of nature.

PLANETARY RULER

Saturn, the planet famous for its intricately structured orbiting rings. Saturn was the Roman god of wealth and agriculture. His counterpart in Greek mythology was Kronos. In astrology, Saturn represents time, limitations, rules, and responsibilities, all integral aspects of the ability to turn ideas into reality.

ELEMENT

Earth, which embodies the grounded energy of creativity, resistance, and practicality. It is fertile and passive, and it relates to the world on a sensual level. Pragmatism, routines, and sensuality energizes earth signs while fast movement, quick change, and an emphasis on sentimentality may deplete their vitality.

MODALITY

Cardinal, which loves beginnings and the first stage of a creative project. Cardinal signs are motivated, ambitious, and enterprising. They encounter stress when things are not fresh and new.

Personal Health Profile

Capricorns thrive on accomplishing goals. So if you set wellness as one of your aims, you'll strive hard to achieve it. With ardent strength in the face of adversity, you are not likely to complain about your health or any aches and pains you may feel. While others may try to elicit sympathy when sick, not Capricorns, whose self-reliant nature likes to maintain a sense of public composure. This may work well to help you power through the limitations that would stop others. Yet a great source of your personal healing can come from knowing that sometimes other people's knowledge and experience can benefit you and that asking for help isn't necessarily a sign of weakness.

As Capricorns don't like to sway much from tradition, when it comes to health care, you're more inclined to follow mainstream, society-sanctioned approaches that boast long, successful track records and a litany of research-based benefits. It's not that you won't try alternative wellness therapies; it's just that you are not the first jumping on the bandwagon of the newest trends. Yet, once you have tried a new natural remedy or therapy and find that it works well for you, you will readily include it as an integral part of your wellness regimen. After all, loyalty is one of the hallmarks of your astrological sign.

Frugal Capricorns should realize that it's possible to be budget conscious and health conscious at the same time. Some of the best things in life, and health care, are free (including stress-relieving techniques such as exercise and meditation) or relatively low cost (such as a whole foods diet). Many insurance companies also offer wellness therapy benefits for

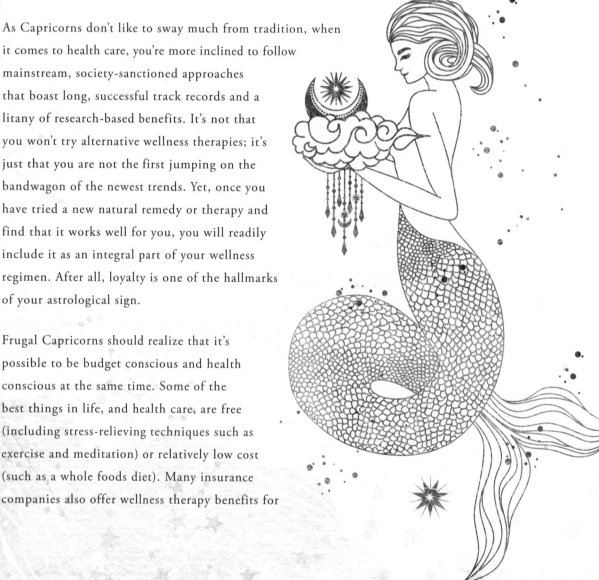

massage, chiropractic, and acupuncture, so out-of-pocket expenses for these services may be minimal. Remember the old maxim, "An ounce of prevention is worth a pound of cure," as it certainly aligns with your conservation-oriented sensibilities.

With your planetary ruler, Saturn, representing limitations and delays, many Capricorns find that life is challenging until they reach their forties, a time when they gracefully hit their stride. It's as if all that hard work you did in your early adulthood finally pays off, with a youthful sense of maturity as the prize.

 ## Areas of Health Focus

The parts of the body associated with Capricorn include:

- The **skeletal system**—including the **bones**, **cartilage**, and **teeth**—that provide you with structure

- The **joints**, in general, and the **knees**, in particular, the bending of which is integral to your ability to move forward in the world

- The **skin**, the protective barrier that encompasses and defines your form

Your Capricornian persistence, strategic approach to getting things accomplished, and committed work ethic are some of the resources you can use when facing any health challenge.

HONOR YOUR KNEES' NEEDS

The sign of Capricorn is associated with the joints, the strength and flexibility of which allow you to confidently move about in your life. As such, you may want to take special care of your joints—especially your knees—to ward off the potential for developing arthritis. Characterized by cartilage and synovial membrane degeneration, arthritis can lead to pain, swelling, and restricted movement. An anti-inflammatory diet—filled with foods and spices rich in omega-3 fatty acids and antioxidants—can do wonders for supporting rheumatoid health, as can watching your stress levels. And speaking of stress, the knees have to support a force equal to two to three times your body weight; therefore, shedding any excess pounds (kilograms) can help reduce the risk of experiencing arthritis in this Capricorn-ruled joint.

SUPPORT SKIN HEALTH

The structure and integrity of the skin is under the auspices of your sign. As such, it may be an area of vulnerability, making it even more important to take extra good care of your skin, protecting it against dryness, breakouts, and rashes. A practical approach to skin health involves following a supportive diet that includes antioxidant-rich fruits and vegetables, omega-3-rich fish and seeds, and filtered water. Investigating whether common food allergens, like dairy and wheat, are contributing to any skin problems (such as dermatitis or acne) you may have is also a good strategy. Additionally, watch out for topical allergies that can be provoked by everyday products such as lotions, cleansers, and laundry detergents.

AVOID BURNOUT

Even though your sign is known for its endurance, Capricorns tend to work so hard pursuing their objectives that they risk running themselves into the ground. As an earth sign, you do have an incredible storehouse of physical resources. Yet, like any other inventory, if it's not replenished, there's a chance you can deplete your stock. If you don't acknowledge your limits, your body will just do it for you, using a cold or other illness as a signal to make you stop and rest. Be proactive and build relaxation time into your schedule. This will make your work life—as well as the rest of your life—more productive and enjoyable.

WORK ON REDUCING ANXIETY

Capricorns take their careers and contributions to society very seriously. You invest great effort in whatever you do, priding yourself on your reputation and how the world sees you. But, as the taskmasters of the zodiac, if you don't feel that you're measuring up to your high ideals, you may descend into feelings of depression or anxiety. If your work isn't working for your mental health, it may be time to retool your attitude and approach. For example, make sure that your aims can be realistically attained in the time frame envisioned. Also, survey your goals and see whether they truly yield personal satisfaction or just fulfill someone else's desires for your life.

Healthy Eating Tips

As someone who cherishes the rules of the natural world, Capricorn will do best with whole foods that provide the nutrients the body needs to function optimally—and therefore, for health to flourish.

MAKE HEALTHY EATING A TOP PRIORITY

As an earth sign, Capricorns are well connected to their bodies, including their sense of hunger and need for nourishment. Yet if you become engrossed in a project—no matter how big or small—you may ignore your appetite and put off eating. If this means meals are delayed a few minutes, that's not a problem. But when it verges on hours, it can wreak havoc on your blood sugar and compromise your sense of well-being. Remember that keeping yourself well nourished is just as important as any other project that captures your attention. Keep nuts, trail mix, or energy bars at your desk or in your car as a time-saving way to keep your energy on track during your busy days.

BONE UP ON A HEALTHY DIET

In addition to dairy products, some of the foods most concentrated in bone-building nutrients—including calcium and magnesium—are green vegetables. They also contain a lot of vitamin K; another rich source of this salutary nutrient is natto, Japanese fermented soybeans, which has been found to be a star food when it comes to preventing bone loss. As important as what to eat is what not to eat: limit caffeine, refined sugar, and salt, as excess may leach calcium from bones, weakening its structural matrix. As a stand-in for coffee, consider drinking green tea. Not only does it have about one-fourth the caffeine, but research suggests that its catechin phytonutrients, notably EGCG, can help increase bone mineral density.

DRINK WATER

Capricorns are often bad at drinking enough water. Why? It's probably the same reason you put off eating—you don't want to divert your attention from the activity at hand. Yet it only takes seconds to sip water, a great investment of time that will yield numerous health benefits. Not only will it improve the tone of your skin, and the strength of your joints, but it is also elemental to good digestion. To save yourself time going to the sink or watercooler, fill up a few bottles in the morning and keep them at your desk (room temperature water is better for your digestion anyway). Look for stainless-steel or glass water bottles, including ones that allow you to infuse the water with fresh herbs.

Health-Supporting Foods

Goats can incorporate many delicious foods into their diets to help promote the health of their Capricorn-ruled bones. These include goat's milk, leafy green vegetables, and foods rich in vitamin D, such as salmon and sardines.

GOAT'S MILK

Unsurprisingly, goat's milk—and the yogurt and cheese made from it—can be a health-supporting food for the Goat. It is rich in calcium, with 1 cup (250 ml) providing over 300 milligrams of this bone-building mineral. Take note if you have dairy allergies: many people who can't tolerate cow's milk do just fine with goat's milk. Goat cheese (also known as chèvre) makes a great addition to salads, sandwiches, and cheese plates. While goat cheese is readily available, goat's milk and yogurt may be more difficult to find in supermarkets. Natural food stores and farmers' markets are usually your best bets for these tart and refreshing foods.

LEAFY GREENS

While leafy greens appear delicate, they can actually form the backbone of a diet that supports Capricorn-ruled bones. Not only do these greens—such as kale, chard, spinach, and collard greens—contain large amounts of calcium, but unlike dairy products, they're also concentrated in bone-strengthening nutrients such as magnesium, vitamin K, and manganese. Additionally, with their abundance of antioxidants that fight cartilage-damaging free radicals, they can make a great contribution to joint health. While it's true that leafy greens contain oxalic acid, the ability of this compound to inhibit calcium absorption is actually minimal. Quickly steaming greens—for not more than five minutes—will help retain many nutrients that would otherwise be lost to overcooking.

VITAMIN D-RICH FOODS

Vitamin D has long been heralded for benefiting Capricorn-ruled bones, with a deficiency of this important nutrient linked to osteoporosis. Recently, vitamin D has also shown health-promoting promise for hypertension, diabetes, depression, and multiple sclerosis. While sun exposure produces vitamin D in the body, ensuring you get adequate amounts through your diet is important. This is notably true for hardworking Capricorns, who, often tied to their desks, may not see the light of day nearly enough. Fish such as salmon, cod, sardines, and mackerel are some of the richest sources of vitamin D. Cow's milk is fortified with this sunshine nutrient as well, although cheese and yogurt generally are not. If your diet doesn't provide you with enough vitamin D, consider taking it in supplement form.

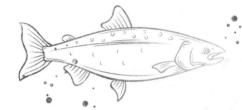

 # Wellness Therapies

Don't let Capricorn frugality stop you from enjoying wellness therapies, especially because they are great investments for your health.

SWEDISH MASSAGE

A Capricorn likes things that function well: easy access and a proven track record are a plus; exotic bells and whistles, not so much. Therefore, Swedish massage—the classic form offered at most spas and health clinics—may serve well as the bodywork of choice for a pragmatic Capricorn. Swedish massage relieves stress and muscular tension as well as symptoms—such as pain and reduced range of motion—associated with arthritis of the Capricorn-ruled knee joint. To get the most from a massage, temper your normal Capricornian reserve and communicate to the practitioner what your body needs and the amount of pressure that feels best.

BODY-MOISTURIZING TREATMENTS

If you're looking to keep your skin healthy and well hydrated, body-moisturizing treatments can make a great addition to your wellness portfolio. These treatments usually begin with exfoliation, a step that preps your skin to absorb moisture both during and afterward. Then a deeply hydrating body mask is applied. Some spas even offer body-moisturizing treatments made from goat's milk, an uber-Capricornian treat. For an at-home approach, apply a deeply nourishing body lotion after scrubbing your body with a loofah or dry brush. An everyday routine of cleansing and moisturizing will also keep your skin in tip-top shape.

FELDENKRAIS METHOD

Ingrained movement patterns—even the ones of a typically efficient Capricorn—often cause wear and tear on the body, manifesting in pain and muscular tension. The Feldenkrais Method is a style of body-awareness training that makes you more conscious of any habitual movement patterns that may not best serve your body's structure and function. Using verbal and light-touch cues, Feldenkrais practitioners teach you to move more efficaciously, allowing you to enjoy reduced strain and increased range of motion. Feldenkrais is available in individual and group sessions. To find a practitioner near you, inquire within your social network, do an online search, or see whether anyone at your gym or yoga studio knows someone trained in this movement-awareness method.

 # Relaxation Practices

For optimal health, Capricorns should work hard at incorporating more relaxation into their schedule.

HIKING

Emanate your astrological totem and climb a mountain (or even just a hill). Hiking is a great way to get some exercise, enjoy the fresh air, and get in touch with nature. If the weather is too inclement for a hike, don't despair; there's always the gym's stair-stepping machine or inclined elliptical trainer when you want an activity that allows you to ascend, albeit virtually, a mountain. Also try out the bouldering wall at a rock-climbing gym to see if that piques your interest. Don't forget that you needn't climb any mountain (literally or figuratively) alone. Consider hiking with a partner, especially if you're concerned about safety.

LABYRINTH WALKING

Walking a labyrinth is a moving meditation with a destination, a differentiation that Capricorns will appreciate. The outward goal—to weave your way through the maze-like structure—naturally reinforces the inner goals of calming your mind and relaxing your body. Knowing that labyrinths are not a New Age creation but a time-honored tradition—the oldest, located on the island of Crete, is more than four thousand years old—will appeal to legacy-honoring Capricorns. Labyrinths can be found throughout the world; cathedrals, public parks, and healing centers are just some of the places that feature these meditative mandalas. If you find these mazes to be amazing for your peace of mind, you can even consider building a simple one in your yard.

FROLIC AND PLAY

All work and no play makes Jack a dull boy (and Jill a dull girl). While you're filling out your calendar with all of your tasks, projects, and deadlines, don't forget to schedule in some fun. While it may seem that you will achieve nothing by playing, a life that has levity and joy is, in itself, a great accomplishment that provides many rewards. Release your inner child and head to the playground. Have fun and relieve stress by swinging on the swings, balancing on the seesaw, and descending the slide with reckless—but careful—abandon.

 # Natural Remedies

Natural remedies can be a very smart and cost-effective way to promote wellness for Capricorns, who appreciate intelligence and a great value.

TURMERIC

Since turmeric has an amazing array of health benefits, practical Capricorns would do well to add it to their medicine (or spice) cabinet. Abundant in the powerful antioxidant and anti-inflammatory compound curcumin, turmeric has been used in Ayurvedic and other traditional medical approaches to treat arthritis. Applied topically, turmeric-infused creams may also help heal skin wounds. While turmeric is available as a dietary supplement in capsule form, you can also buy the powdered spice or fresh root at your market and incorporate it into recipes. Be careful when using it, though: while it can have an indelibly positive effect on your health, turmeric can also create an indelible stain on your clothes (and sometimes a temporary one on your skin).

GLUCOSAMINE SULFATE

Glucosamine sulfate is one of the most popular dietary supplements for relieving the symptoms of arthritis and improving the overall health of the Capricorn-ruled knees. Since it is a precursor of cartilage molecules, glucosamine strengthens this connective tissue rather than just providing symptomatic relief like many over-the-counter anti-inflammatory medicines do. Several research studies have found glucosamine sulfate reduces joint stiffness and pain. If you're watching your salt intake, look for glucosamine stabilized with potassium sulfate rather than sodium sulfate. Those with diabetes may want to check with their doctors before taking glucosamine because there's a possibility that the supplement can elevate blood sugar levels.

S-ADENOSYLMETHIONINE (*SAMe*)

SAMe (pronounced "SAM-mee") is a naturally occurring compound derived from methionine, one of the only two food-based amino acids that contain sulfur, a mineral associated with your planetary ruler, Saturn. SAMe's claim to fame is that it is one of the best methyl donors around, and because methylation is critical to so many body functions, its benefits are widespread. SAMe is thought to hold promise for alleviating health conditions such as arthritis and depression, as well as discouraging age-related cognitive decline. It's best to take SAMe during the day as it may give you an energy boost that could inhibit sound sleep if you take it too close to bedtime.

 # Essential Oils

Aromatherapy embraces qualities elemental to a Capricorn because it is an easy-to-use, relatively inexpensive, and readily accessible wellness practice.

CYPRESS (*CUPRESSUS SEMPERVIRENS*)

The Saturn-ruled cypress tree is so strong that its wood was prized in antiquity and used to construct ships and buildings. The fortitude of its essential oil, distilled from its leaves, is also well known in its own right. Especially good for soothing rheumatic pain and enhancing skin tone, cypress can inspire calm in a Capricorn during times of grief and crisis. To use, soak a small towel in a mixture of cypress and warm water, applying it as a compress to sore joints. During times of emotional upheaval, keep a cypress-scented handkerchief with you so you can readily inhale its soothing aroma.

FRANKINCENSE (*BOSWELLIA* SPP.)

Frankincense has great skin-rejuvenating properties, an especially beneficial attribute for Capricorns, and a quality well regarded by the ancient Egyptians, who utilized it in their cosmetics. It can also be used for easing rheumatic pain. Not only valued for its practical uses, frankincense is also endowed with inspirational properties; it was one of the gifts of the magi, after all, and is commonly used in religious rites as well. As a balm for achy joints, add some frankincense to unscented massage oil. You can also mix a drop or two into your moisturizer to enhance skin tone. Burning frankincense resin over incense charcoal can add a divine fragrance to your environment.

SCOTCH PINE (*PINUS SYLVESTRIS*)

Scotch pine is a great scent to use all year long, but especially during the winter season, when the forest aroma of this oil can create a warming atmosphere. It kills fungus and other microbes that can compromise your home's air quality, a notable benefit when the cold weather keeps you indoors. Additionally, it's thought to enhance circulation and help battle respiratory infections, with an exhilarating scent that's just the ticket for lifting the winter blues. You can use Scotch pine essential oil in an aromatherapy diffuser to freshen the air. Blend with massage oil for a vitalizing muscle-relaxing treatment (but test on a small patch of skin first, as some people find that it irritates their skin).

 ## Flower Essences

Once a down-to-earth Capricorn sees how effective flower essences are at balancing emotional and psychological well-being, these remedies will become a regularly relied-upon facet of your wellness regimen. (See page 20 for how to use flower essences.)

OAK (*QUERCUS ROBUR*)

Capricorns are the masters of burning the candle at both ends; this may lead to your great productivity and yet it can put you at risk for burnout. While you set your sights high on all you want to achieve for yourself and those you love, it's important for you to realize that, in fact, one person is only capable of doing so much. Oak flower essence can help you gracefully surrender to your limits and more readily ask for assistance from others. It can prove a great stress reliever, helping diminish a tendency toward placing unrelenting demands on yourself.

MIMULUS (*MIMULUS GUTTATUS*)

Capricorns hold themselves to very high standards. The idea of failure—of not attaining one's sought-after goals—is one of the Goat's greatest fears. While you may be inclined to use this fear of failure as motivation, it can also undermine your ability to make objective judgments, compelling you to act from an emotional, rather than a rational, space. Mimulus is an effective flower essence for inspiring courage and confidence, which, when partnered with your perseverance, is an unbeatable combination.

VINE (*VITIS VINIFERA*)

Confident Capricorns would rather lead than follow, knowing that they can get the job done right. Yet keep in mind that too much persistent self-reliance can sometimes lead to a myopic vision of what others are capable of and the importance of their unique contributions. Vine flower essence is a good remedy to use when you need a reminder that delegating is not the sign of a weak leader but a powerful one who successfully empowers others.

 # Yoga Poses

Yoga can be a pragmatic way for a Capricorn to gain strength and flexibility. Look for a teacher who focuses on alignment to best safeguard joint health.

MOUNTAIN (*TADASANA*)

Mastering Mountain pose—a basic yoga posture that focuses on alignment and solidity—can help the Goat reach the top of any peak.

- Stand with your feet together or hip-width apart, whichever feels better, with your weight evenly distributed through your feet. Lift your kneecaps by engaging your

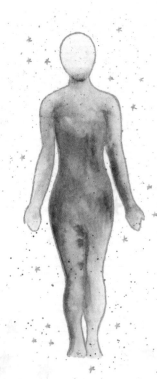

quadriceps muscles, while you also lift the muscles of your pelvic floor in and up toward your navel. Squeeze your shoulder blades into your back, widen across the front of your chest, and rest your arms at your sides. The crown of your head should float above the center of your body, and you should feel a strong line of energy from your feet all the way to the top of your head. Stay in the pose for up to one minute.

CHAIR (*UTKATASANA*)

Not only does the bending involved in Chair pose promote flexibility and range of motion, but it also strengthens the quadriceps muscles, supporting proper alignment of the Capricorn-ruled kneecaps.

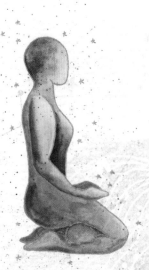

- Stand in Mountain pose (see previous description). Raise your arms overhead, with your palms facing each other. Slowly bend your knees until your thighs are almost parallel to the ground. Keep your spine long as you sit down and back, keeping your feet grounded into the floor. Your torso will naturally lean forward so that your body is in a somewhat zigzag position. Stay in the pose for up to one minute.

HERO (*VIRASANA*)

Known for their many achievements and valiant characteristics, Capricorns definitely embody heroic tendencies. Hero pose is a great posture to bring flexibility to your knee and ankle joints.

- Kneel on the floor, with your knees parallel and your shins angling out, so your feet are positioned wider than your hips. Rest the top of your ankles on the floor (if this position is painful, place a block under your hips or a rolled-up blanket under your ankles or knees). Slowly begin to sit back between your feet. As you do so, place

Inspiring Sleep

With your achievement orientation, a Capricorn may feel that sleep is an unwelcome distraction to being productive and getting things accomplished. Yet, the opposite is actually true. Good sleep is associated with better concentration, enhanced memory, and greater productivity—all keys to the success you value. You can also use the power of your dreaming mind to discover sought-after work solutions by practicing dream incubation (see page 238).

your hands on your upper calves, and gently move your muscles to the outside to avoid compressing them. Point your feet straight back and not out to the sides. Sit up tall, maintaining a sense of inner lift while relaxing your neck and shoulders. Stay in the pose for up to one minute at first, gradually working your way up to five minutes.

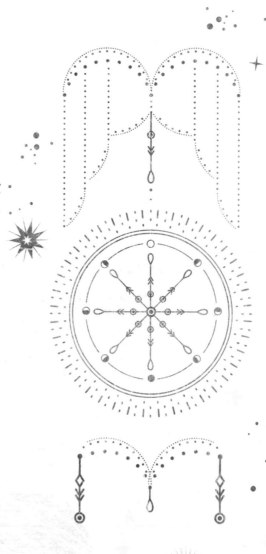

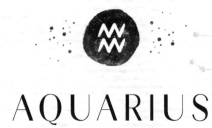

AQUARIUS

CHARACTERISTICS

Altruistic, cerebral, detached, eccentric, egalitarian, friendly, independent, innovative, perceptive, philanthropic, progressive, rebellious.

SYMBOL

The Water Bearer, a figure who gathers wisdom and insight, offering it in service to the world. In mythological traditions, the Water Bearer sustains and advances life on Earth.

PLANETARY RULER

Uranus, known for its unique orbit. Uranus was the Greek god of the sky. His counterpart in Roman mythology was Caelus. In astrology, Uranus represents innovation, sudden revelations, rebellion, and creative chaos. Saturn—representing time, limitations, and rules—is this sign's traditional ruler.

ELEMENT

Air, which is associated with the agile energy of thoughts, observation, and logic. It is social, intellectual, changeable, and relationship oriented. Mental activities, communicating, and creating alliances energizes air signs while stasis, too much practicality, and heightened emotionality may deplete their vitality.

MODALITY

Fixed, which adores the planning and building phase of a creative project. Fixed signs prize reliability, predictability, and stamina. Discontinuity or too much change may throw them off their A-game.

161

Personal Health Profile

Aquarius is a sign that embodies great vitality. You maintain a dynamic energy and sense of composure that can translate into sustained good health.

Physical ailments generally seem to bother you less than they do others. That's partially a result of your Aquarian altruistic nature: you are simply less concerned with yourself than about the welfare of others. It is also because, as an air sign, Aquarius are not as rooted in their bodies, living more in their highly perceptive minds. Yet, you can use this proclivity to your health advantage; for example, pay attention to any out-of-the-blue flashes of insight—which Aquarius regularly experiences—that have to do with your well-being.

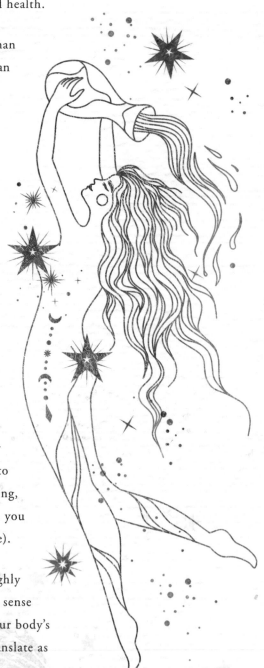

As a global citizen, you don't discriminate based on origins and are equally comfortable with those who come from across the ocean as down the street. This respect for other cultures may translate into a wellness regimen that resembles the United Nations: for example, essential oils from India, herbs and spices from the Middle East, and relaxation practices from China. With a keen ability to perceive vibrations, you're likely to be attracted to energy medicine: while acupuncture, hands-on healing, and flower essences may seem "New Agey" to some, you tend to consider them timeless (and highly effective).

This openness to energy is also reflected in your highly charged internal circuitry and heightened ability to sense electromagnetic fields. Therefore, disruptions in your body's bioelectrical system (including your "aura") may translate as low-level interruptions in your sense of wellness, possibly experienced as energy depletion, irritability, and frazzled nerves. These disruptions may be caused by overexposure to the computers, cell phones, and other technological wizardry so ubiquitous in the modern world (and to which many Water Bearers are so attracted). For optimal Aquarian health, it's important to pull the plug on the information superhighway every now and then to keep your own internal circuitry humming properly.

Rebels at heart, Aquarius are not ones to submit to society-sanctioned authorities and, as such, many Water Bearers are equally comfortable getting their wellness needs met by an acupuncturist or naturopathic physician as they are by a conventional medical doctor. Whichever type of health-care practitioner you choose, look for one who can see you as the complex and integrated individual that you are.

 ## Areas of Health Focus

The parts of the body associated with Aquarius include:

- The **lower legs**, including the **calf muscles**, **Achilles tendon**, and **peripheral circulatory system**
- The **ankles**, the flexibility and structure of which allow for efficient movement
- The **retina** of the eye, which provides you with vision
- The **bioelectrical system**, the electromagnetic waves inherent in, and radiating from, all body cells

Your Aquarian keen mind, strong intuitive awareness, and ability to see the big picture are some of the resources you can use when facing any health challenge.

MIND YOUR LOWER LEGS AND ANKLES

Aquarius have some things in connection with the Greek hero Achilles. You're both fearless warriors committed to fighting for their cause and a spot of vulnerability for you is the eponymous tendon named after him (as well as the rest of your lower leg, including your calf and ankle). Numerous afflictions can impact this area of the body, including muscles spasms, shin splints, restless legs syndrome, and swollen or twisted ankles. As Aquarius are prone to experiencing the unexpected, take extra precautions when exercising to guard against injury. As for your diet, magnesium- and potassium-rich foods, including fruits and vegetables, can help keep your muscles functioning smoothly.

PREVENT VARICOSE VEINS

Your sign's rebellious nature extends to the workings of the body as well, with Aquarius ruling physiological actions that go against the natural gradient. One such example is peripheral blood circulation, notably the action of the Aquarius-ruled calves to pump blood back from the lower body to the heart in an action that defies gravity. If this function isn't working properly, it can manifest in varicose veins. While a doctor should be consulted to rule out the more serious chronic venous insufficiency condition that can compromise overall health, there are some general self-care treatments that can benefit your legs. For example, walk regularly to stimulate circulation, apply a compress of witch hazel to your calves, and consider vein-strengthening herbs such as butcher's broom (see page 170), horse chestnut, and gotu kola.

PROTECT YOUR VISION

Aquarius are visionaries, blessed with an ability to sense a cohesive pattern and see how pathways rooted in the present world can lead to a more altruistic future. Your sign is also associated with vision—the sense of sight, that is—because it not only governs the retina but also the process of perceiving and translating light waves into images. You can take care of your eyes by wearing UV-ray-blocking sunglasses and eating a diet that includes fish, carotenoid-rich fruits and vegetables, and leafy greens. A good multivitamin can also help cover all your bases when it comes to the numerous nutrients that support optimal eye health.

RECHARGE YOUR INTERNAL CIRCUITRY

Aquarius possess a large sensory radar screen, which allows them to perceive a greater degree of stimuli, including subtle energies and vibrations. While this gives you access to greater perceptions than most, it may also overtax your nervous system at times, which may lead to feelings of restlessness, anxiety, and exhaustion. To pacify your internal circuitry, take time away from technology every once in a while (for example, make Sunday a day of rest from the computer). Spending time outdoors can also help you resonate with the more harmonious vibrations of nature. Additionally, a whole-foods diet can benefit the nervous system, with several nutrients—including omega-3 fats, vitamin B6, and folate—playing especially important roles in promoting nerve health.

 # Healthy Eating Tips

Less in their bodies than in their minds, Aquarius need to ensure that they don't overlook the importance of a healthy diet for their physical and mental well-being.

HONOR YOUR NEED FOR FREEDOM

You cherish your liberty; as an Aquarius, you desire to be free to do what you want when you want. This includes eating. While others may subscribe to a regular routine, eating according to expectations goes against your independent nature. So honor the nonconformist in you and eat to the beat of your own mealtime drum. Give yourself the freedom to eat when it seems right to do so. While Aquarius are not always in tune with what *feels* nourishing for their bodies, use your perceptive mind to *know* what would be nurturing; look for signs and signals—such as if your nervous system feels a bit frayed—that will help you tailor your meal patterns.

EAT RAW AND GROUNDING FOODS

Eating fresh, raw foods keeps Aquarius buzzing, providing you with the life-force energy that helps your mind stay resonant and astutely aware of the subtleties of your environment. Yet an overreliance on raw foods can make you feel ungrounded. The solution: eat fruit, enjoy vegetables in both their raw and lightly cooked forms, and include a range of grounding foods such as nuts, beans, and whole grains in your diet. An easy way to ensure you're eating fresh, raw foods is to enjoy a salad at lunch and/or dinner. Quickly cooking vegetables—most can be steamed in five minutes or less—preserves nutrients. It also saves time, a plus for an Aquarius, as you would rather be out saving the world than spending extra time in the kitchen.

CHOOSE FOODS THAT BENEFIT CIRCULATION

Because Aquarius is associated with the peripheral circulatory system and the lower legs, eating a diet to promote the integrity of your veins and capillaries is central to elevating your health. While all nutrients are important, antioxidants—including vitamins C and E as well as flavonoid phytonutrients—are particularly beneficial when it comes to buttressing blood vessels and avoiding varicose veins. While most people think of oranges as the premier source of vitamin C, guavas, strawberries, papaya, and kiwifruit actually contain more of it on a per calorie basis. Sunflower seeds, almonds, mustard greens, and olives are all rich in vitamin E. And any time you see a purple- or red-colored fruit or vegetable, it is a good bet that it is filled with flavonoids.

Health-Supporting Foods

There are many foods Aquarius can choose to help them sustain their energetic stability. Some beneficial ones for the Water Bearer include exotic fruit, green tea, and lutein- and zeaxanthin-rich foods.

EXOTIC FRUIT

Aquarius are the global citizens of the zodiac, and as such, they find the exotic both attractive and familiar. That's of benefit when it comes to fruits from other cultures—such as goji and acai berries, and even the more common papaya and pineapple—which can be health-promoting additions to an Aquarian diet. Goji berries are rich in vision-promoting carotenoid phytonutrients and can be enjoyed as part of an energy-boosting trail mix. Anthocyanin-rich acai is available in juice form as well as in frozen packs that you can add to smoothies. In addition to the numerous vitamins and minerals they contain, papaya and pineapple are rich in digestion-enhancing enzymes.

GREEN TEA

Oscillating Aquarius likes the buzz that caffeine provides. Yet too much caffeine—the amount provided by just two medium cups of coffee—can have a diuretic effect, pulling vital water from your body. So after your first cup of coffee, consider switching to antioxidant-rich green tea. It features less than half the caffeine, yet it can provide you with steady energy throughout the day. Green tea comes in many different varieties; the most popular are sencha, hojicha, bancha, and genmaicha. When making green tea, don't use boiling water—a below-simmer 165°–175°F (75°–80°C), depending upon variety, should be the maximum.

LUTEIN- AND ZEAXANTHIN-RICH FOODS

Lutein and zeaxanthin are related antioxidant carotenoid phytonutrients found concentrated in yellow-colored foods, such as corn, winter squash, and egg yolks, as well as in deep green leafy vegetables. They can also be found in the retina and lens of your eyes, where they protect against Sun-induced damage. Eating foods rich in these phytonutrients can help reduce your risk of developing cataracts and macular degeneration. To amplify your intake of these nutrients, add spinach to an omelet for a colorful and delicious breakfast. With its sweet flavor, winter squash makes a great side dish; cut into small cubes, it steams in less than ten minutes. While fresh corn is nutrient-rich, products made from it—such as corn oil and high-fructose corn syrup—are not.

 # Wellness Therapies

With their global perspective and open-mindedness, Aquarius appreciate how wellness treatments from other cultures can be of great benefit.

ACUPUNCTURE

The Water Bearer will consider the virtue of a wellness technique even if it hasn't passed muster with society's traditional methods of assessing efficacy. Take acupuncture, for example, a system of healing that has yet to be "proven" by Western science but one whose inherent value the Aquarian mind can perceive. Acupuncture also speaks to your awareness that even if something is imperceptible, that doesn't mean it doesn't exist: the fact that health can be attained through balancing *chi* (subtle energy) by inserting needles along the body's invisible energy meridians seems as "real" to an Aquarius as anything else.

REIKI

Another wellness therapy that focuses on balancing vital energy is reiki (pronounced RAY-kee), a type of hands-on healing practice. While meditating on different symbols, the practitioner transmits *chi* (life force energy), which the recipient experiences as a warm flow of radiant energy. Reiki is great for stress reduction and relaxation, and may also help relieve chronic pain. Some practitioners offer distance reiki sessions, in which you don't need to be in the same physical space to have a treatment. If you like the experience of receiving reiki, consider training in this healing method, as it can be a great way to further connect with your own energy.

NIA TECHNIQUE

As an Aquarius, you thrive in group situations that allow you to express your freedom and individuality. That's why the NIA technique—an eclectic fitness system that's a combination of dance, martial arts, yoga, and movement therapy—is so well suited to your nature. NIA classes provide a flexible structure in which each participant has the autonomy to guide their own individual movement experiences. NIA not only tones and strengthen muscles and joints, but it also provides an energizing approach to balancing the nervous system. NIA classes are taught at spas, fitness centers, and dance studios. You can also stream classes online if you want to do an at-home workout.

 # Relaxation Practices

It is important for Water Bearers to take time to recharge their batteries every now and again with activities that nurture both mind and body.

QIGONG

Qigong is a meditative movement practice that has many Aquarian characteristics, including an egalitarian- and community-oriented nature; for example, in its native land of China, young and old, rich and poor, take part in qigong, with large classes occurring in public outdoor spaces. During this practice, you perform gentle movements that open your awareness to vibrational fields within and around you. You also hone in on your sensory perception, which can become sharper and more precise over time. There are numerous qigong books and videos available that describe the fundamentals of this mindfulness practice. Although you can practice qigong on your own, it is best to first learn proper techniques from a skilled teacher in a class setting.

MINERAL SALT BATH

The symbol for Aquarius is the Water Bearer, a figure who pours this life-sustaining liquid from an urn, offering it in service to humanity. Gift yourself the benefits of this vital elixir by regularly soaking in a hot bath. Water infused with minerals, such as magnesium-containing Epsom salts, will relax your muscles and improve your circulation. Salt is said to harmonize a person's energy field, a benefit for electronically sensitive Aquarius. In addition to Epsom salts, you can purchase salts derived from the Dead Sea or Himalayan regions, which feature a different mixture of minerals. For additional healing, add aromatherapy oils or flower essences to the bath.

VOLUNTEERING

At the heart of the Aquarian nature is the desire to make a difference, to help better the world. Yet to do so, you don't want to go it alone; rather, as a socially oriented person, you appreciate being part of a collective of like-minded individuals. For an activity that fulfills your altruistic spirit and leaves you feeling more harmonious, consider doing public service work. Volunteering at a food bank, fund-raising for your favorite charity, or advocating for the rights of the underprivileged are just a few of the numerous ways you can contribute to your community, near or far. Look for websites that will match your interests, skills, and geographic location to available public service opportunities.

 # Natural Remedies

As a trendsetting Aquarius, you probably used natural remedies long before they became popular.

SIBERIAN GINSENG (*ELEUTHEROCOCCUS SENTICOSUS*)

One of your planetary rulers, Uranus, symbolizes unpredictability. While you are used to expecting the unexpected, even the perceptive Aquarius gets caught off guard by stress and trauma. Siberian ginseng can help increase the body's resistance to stresses—whether they be physical, electromagnetic, or chemical—that may otherwise deplete energy. It is used to increase mental focus, physical endurance, and immune-system function as well as to protect against stress-related illnesses. Also known as eleuthero, Siberian ginseng is available in dried herb, capsule, or liquid tincture form. Because of its energy-boosting effects, it should not be taken close to bedtime.

BUTCHER'S BROOM (*RUSCUS ACULEATUS*)

If you want to sweep away obstacles that may keep you from optimal health—notably if lower leg health is a concern—try butcher's broom. This saponin-rich herb has been found to be an effective remedy for many people experiencing varicose veins, helping to relieve the leg pain and swelling associated with this condition. Butcher's broom improves sluggish lower-leg circulation by supporting the integrity of the veins as well as combating inflammation. It is available in capsule and liquid tincture forms. Research has found that vitamin C supports the effectiveness of butcher's broom, so consider supplementing with this nutrient as well.

PASSIONFLOWER (*PASSIFLORA INCARNATA*)

If you are looking for a natural way to induce calm when you're feeling a bit buzzy and ramped up, you might develop a passion for his herbal remedy. You can take passionflower on its own, although it is often found in botanical combination formulas with other sedative herbs, including skullcap and hops. Passionflower is available in dried herb, capsule, and liquid tincture form. It also comes in a homeopathic version, known as passiflora. Mint and coffee can counteract the effectiveness of homeopathic remedies, so avoid them for several hours before and after taking passiflora.

 # Essential Oils

The fragrant scents of essential oils can help progressive and globally focused Water Bearers feel more rooted in their bodies.

PATCHOULI (*POGOSTEMON CABLIN*)

Patchouli is one of the scents most associated with the 1960s, conjuring images of that era's free-spiritedness, mirroring the essence of Aquarius. Yet its redeeming reputation preceded that; in the early nineteenth century, it was included with shipments of fine Indian fabric imported into Europe, where its scent became a symbol of high quality. Patchouli's sweet, musky aroma makes it a grounding aphrodisiac, helping you take root in your body while inspiring openness to sensual pleasure. It is also good for the health of the circulatory system and lower legs. Use it in a room diffuser when you need to feel both grounded and energized. Mix a few drops with some body oil for a tension-freeing and vein-supporting calf massage.

SWEET MARJORAM (*ORIGANUM MAJORANA*)

Sweet marjoram is associated with eternal peace and happiness, quintessential Aquarian ideals. This pacifying herb is known for its antispasmodic and circulation-enhancing properties, traditionally used for a variety of cardiovascular concerns such as high blood pressure. If your nervous system feels particularly overstimulated, sweet marjoram—with its tension-calming effects—may provide the soothing you need. Place a marjoram-scented sachet under your pillow to induce slumber. If muscle cramps—including those in the Aquarius-ruled calves—have you in a bind, apply marjoram-infused massage oil to your legs.

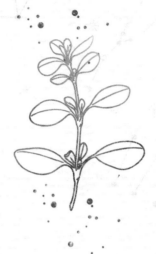

BENZOIN (*STYRAX BENZOIN*)

Burned as incense in the churches and temples of various religions, benzoin is an iconic fragrance signifying spiritual protection. Benzoin is used in perfumery and healing traditions throughout the world and is an equal opportunity remedy that may quiet muscle spasms and support the nervous system. You can also use it for its superior skin-soothing properties. Benzoin is available in a variety of forms, including pure resin, essential oil, and powder. Carry a piece of resin with you, inhaling its uplifting fragrance throughout the day. Add a few drops of essential oil to a bath and enjoy its muscle-relaxing—and numinous—properties.

 # Flower Essences

The fact that a distillation of flowers can deliver psycho-emotional healing doesn't seem odd to an Aquarius, whose out-of-the-box way of thinking may inspire a greater appreciation for the realm of vibrational medicines. (See page 20 for how to use flower essences.)

CALIFORNIA WILD ROSE (*ROSA CALIFORNICA*)

Abetted by their brilliant minds and progressive vision, Aquarius can be of great service to the world when they are aligned with their ideals. Yet sometimes Water Bearers lose sight of their conviction-filled urns. Veiled in apathy, you might feel more like a spectator of life than a participant. When you're feeling a bit isolated and need to reenergize your commitment to your altruistic visions, consider using California Wild Rose.

DILL (*ANETHUM GRAVEOLENS*)

While Water Bearers respect technology's ability to progress society to a higher level, your enhanced consciousness may also make you more open to feeling its subtle effects in your body. To bolster your aura (your personal electromagnetic field) and avoid short-circuiting your nervous system by stimulation overload, consider Dill flower essence. Think of it as a fusible link, helping protect against excess currents that could overwhelm your individual energy system.

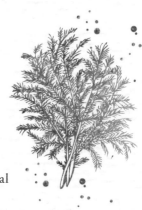

172

QUAKING GRASS (*BRIZA MAXIMA*)

Aquarius are strong individuals who derive much of their identity from belonging to a group. The collective element is important to you because it fosters a much-desired sense of connectivity. Yet feeling at home in a group is not always fun and games, even for the socially minded Aquarius. Quaking Grass flower essence can be used by an individual—as well as members of a group—to help the collective work more harmoniously toward their goals.

 # Yoga Poses

Yoga is a movement practice that lets Aquarius tone their bodies, fortify their life force energy, and exercise their consciousness.

DOWNWARD FACING DOG (*ADHO MUKHA SAVASANA*)

Downward Facing Dog is one of the best poses to bring circulation to the Aquarius-ruled calves and ankles. As you need to focus on many different areas of the body at once during this mild inversion pose, it is particularly well suited to your multifaceted awareness.

- Place your hands and knees on the floor, with your wrists slightly in front of your shoulders and your knees below your hips. Spread your fingers wide, and have your middle finger pointing forward. Curl your toes under, and gently push your knees away from the floor, straightening your legs without locking your knees. Lift your sit bones to the sky, and try to have your heels descend to the floor while lifting your inner ankles. Broaden your shoulder blades. Your head should rest between your arms. Hold the pose for up to one minute.

NOOSE (*PASHASANA*)

Freedom-loving Aquarius doesn't generally like restrictions. But the confines of Noose pose can actually be very liberating to the Water Bearer, because this squatting twist helps stimulate circulation and energy flow, stretches the Achilles tendons, and enhances ankle flexibility.

- Stand with the right side of your body facing the wall, about a forearm's distance away. Gently twist, placing your right palm on the wall while keeping your forearm parallel to the ground. Bend your knees and slowly move into a squatting position (if your heels don't reach the floor, support them with a folded mat or rolled-up blanket). Turning your torso to the right, place your left hand on the wall and your left elbow on the outside of the right knee. Press your elbow and knee together, allowing the resistance to help you twist more deeply so that your torso turns to face the wall. Stay in the pose for up to one minute, and then repeat on the other side. (For the full expression of the pose, practice without the wall.)

Inspiring Sleep

With an avant-garde orientation, Aquarius are often one step ahead of others, including in being early adopters of all things cutting edge. With a confidence to discover innovative solutions, you may find yourself with an affinity to technologies—smart mattresses, wearable devices, and relaxation programs—that can help you hack a better night's sleep. And for Water Bearers interested in their oneiric journeys, apps that connect you to dreamers around the world may offer reward.

RECLINING BIG TOE (*SUPTA PADANGUSTHASANA*)

If you want an asana that helps you stretch the back of your legs without placing stress on your lower back, try Reclining Big Toe pose. It allows you to rest comfortably on the ground, supported by the floor, while you send your leg high into the air, increasing the flexibility of your lower body.

■ Lie on the floor with your legs outstretched. Place a strap around the ball of your right foot; holding the ends of the strap, gently straighten your leg, sending it toward the ceiling. Flex your right foot while keeping your right hip on the floor. (If you have a lot of flexibility, you can do this posture without the aid of the strap by looping your right index and middle fingers around your big toe.) Your left leg should press into the ground, and your left foot should be flexed. If you need more support, bend the left leg, placing your foot on the floor. Stay in the pose for up to one minute, and then repeat on the other side.

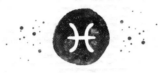

PISCES

CHARACTERISTICS

Dreamy, elusive, empathetic, forgiving, idealistic, imaginative, impressionable, poetic, psychic, selfless, spacey, spiritual.

SYMBOL

A pair of Fish bound together yet swimming in opposite directions, which reflects the mission of integrating the spiritual and material worlds. In mythological and cultural traditions, the Fish is a symbol of unity, sacrifice, transformation, and wisdom.

PLANETARY RULER

Neptune, the planet known for its oceanic blue color. Neptune was the Roman god of the sea. His counterpart in Greek mythology was Poseidon. In astrology, Neptune represents unity, transcendence, and the numinous. Jupiter—representing growth, good fortune, and faith—is this sign's traditional ruler.

ELEMENT

Water, which embraces the fluid energy of emotion, reflection, and nonlinear understanding. It is sensitive, personal, and responsive. Feelings, empathy, and soulful connections energize water signs while excess rationality, lack of personal space, and inability to access their intuition may deplete their vitality.

MODALITY

Mutable, which has an affinity for the adjustment and finessing stage of a creative project. Mutable signs are flexible, adaptive, and chameleon-like. They may find themselves agitated if things are too structured or overly defined.

Personal Health Profile

The symbol for Pisces—two Fish that are swimming in opposite directions—is a great metaphor for the duality inherent in your sign's attitude toward health. One side of the Piscean nature is characterized by an inclination to ignore messages your body is sending you that something's off kilter while the other is typified by a tendency to become overly focused on health and well-being issues. Echoing your sign's propensity for paradox, most Pisces continually float between these two extremes.

The Piscean characteristic of turning a blind eye to health needs reflects your reputation for being the escape artist of the zodiac. As denizens of denial, Pisces will take refuge in daydreams when reality doesn't quite match their idealistic vision of the world. Your dreamy nature often overshadows an ability to feel grounded in, and connected to, your body; as such, you might neglect to notice signs and symptoms of health imbalances. Most Pisces need to be reminded of the importance of staying rooted in their bodies so that they can be conscious of, rather than overlook, their physical needs.

The Fish's opposite inclination is to obsessively fret over matters of health. The Piscean penchant for perfection can make every little itch, bump, or twinge seem like a cause for alarm and a pink slip from good health. Reflecting your sign's dualism, this anxiety-filled focus may cause you to imagine problems where there are none, although it can also

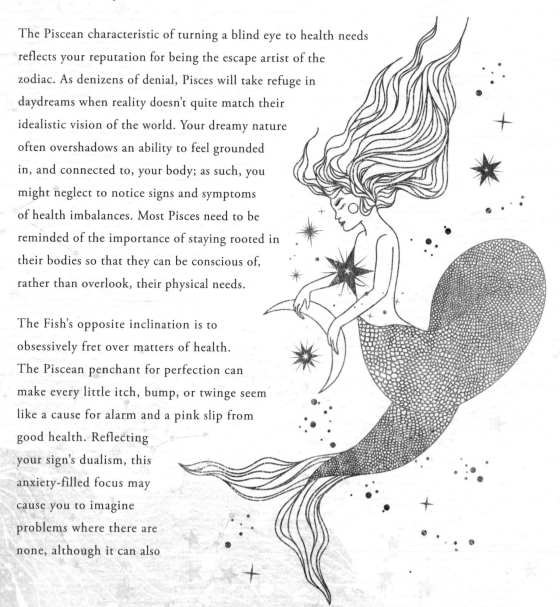

echo an innate sensitivity that enables you to perceive what may be imperceptible to many others. The trick, of course, is to readily discern the cause of your hypochondriacal notions, something that can become more clear through relaxation practices such as meditation, which can help you quiet your mind, tune into your body, and align with your inherent Piscean psychic gifts.

Another Piscean characteristic that influences your attitude toward health is a tendency to experience the world in a more holistic and poetic way than others: where many see separation, you see unity. This is the one reason that Pisces seem especially open to mind-body-spirit approaches to healing. When looking for a health-care practitioner, it's best to find one who is extremely compassionate and honors your high level of sensitivity.

 ## Areas of Health Focus

The parts of the body associated with Pisces include:

- The **feet**, which connect you to the Earth

- The **immune** and **lymphatic systems**, your body's sentries against infection and disease

- The **pineal gland**, which synthesizes the hormone melatonin and is associated with the third eye and heightened psychic abilities in several spiritual traditions

Your Piscean psychic abilities, awareness of the body-mind-spirit connection, and innate sense of compassion are some of the resources you can use when facing any health challenge.

SUPPORT YOUR SOULFUL SOLES

Even when walking down the street, Pisces tend to have their head in the clouds rather than their focus on the ground, leading to a greater than fair share of stubbed toes. Try to put your inclination to daydream on hold while navigating your environment to avoid running into those couches, curbs, and corners that seem to just magically appear. Also, while you may appreciate the glamour of designer shoes, don't sacrifice comfort for fashion; your gentle soles need support—whether in a strappy sandal or winter boot—to avoid the aches and blisters to which they are inclined. If you are prone to athlete's foot, topically applied tea tree oil (see page 185) may do wonders, as can thoroughly drying your feet after bathing or swimming.

BOLSTER YOUR IMMUNE SYSTEM

With your wide-eyed nature and fluid personal boundaries, Pisces often appear more sensitive to outside influences than others. And since bacteria and viruses are no exception, during the change of seasons—or any time you're under undue stress—pay extra attention to fortifying your immune system to protect against colds and flu. To strengthen your defenses, enjoy an array of different nutrient-rich fruits and vegetables throughout the day and consider adding reishi mushrooms (see page 183), vitamin C, and zinc lozenges to your immune-buoying medicine cabinet. As nervous tension can compromise immune system function, meditation and gentle exercise can help shore up your permeable boundaries to keep colds and flu at bay.

GET A GOOD NIGHT'S SLEEP

With one of your planetary rulers, Neptune, governing sleep, getting a good night's rest is especially important for Pisces. It's usually pretty easy for you to dive into slumber the moment your head hits the pillow, but when day-to-day stress rocks your emotional boat, insomnia can become an unwelcome bedfellow. Relaxing essential oils—such as sandalwood (page 184) and myrrh (page 184)—and a little evening meditation can be great tools to help you journey to the land of Nod. Also keep a notebook by your bedside to write down your dreams, a source of great insight for Pisces and an approach more illuminating than counting sheep should you need assistance falling back to sleep.

PROTECT YOUR VITAL ENERGY

While your intensely caring Piscean nature may be one of your greatest gifts, a desire to heal the woes of the world may also be one of your wellness weak spots. You have a tendency to give away a lot of time and space to other people, which can deplete your vital reserves and make you more prone to illness. Because Pisces are so sensitive to others' suffering, they may sometimes even absorb their distress; for example, if your friend has a headache, it may not be uncommon for you to then feel one coming on. It's important to remember that compassion begins at home: concern for your own wellness—as opposed to solely focusing on everyone else's—will allow you to be an altruist without becoming a martyr. Remember, just because Pisces rules the feet does not mean that you have to walk a mile in everyone's shoes.

Healthy Eating Tips

Often more focused on others than self, Pisces need to remember that taking the time to nourish their body and spirit through eating well is inextricably linked to well-being.

EAT CONSCIOUSLY

With a tendency to daydream through many of life's activities (including eating), Pisces can consume a meal in no time flat without even tasting their food or remembering what they ate. Eating consciously is especially beneficial for the Fish, as it can help you feel more grounded in your body. Be mindful when you're eating; savor your food, taking at least fifteen minutes to enjoy each meal. Chew well and relish each bite, paying attention to its taste, texture, and aroma. Not only will this help you feel more satiated, but it will also lessen your chances of experiencing indigestion. Also, before you eat, say a blessing to honor your food to initiate a meal of conscious eating.

STOP DOING THE JITTERBUG

With your heightened sensitivity, life can often be overwhelming for a Pisces. As a coping mechanism, you might rely on caffeine, sugar, and other substances to bolster your mood and energy level. Yet in reality, this strategy is anything but productive, as your impressionable constitution may make you overly susceptible to their stimulating properties. This can exacerbate feelings of spaciness as well as physical and emotional exhaustion. Therefore, think twice before ordering that second latte; instead, enjoy rejuvenating, yet caffeine-free, herbal teas such as rooibos or tulsi. Maple syrup and coconut sugar are nutrient-rich alternatives to refined sugar, while stevia adds sweetness without calories.

LIMIT THE LIBATIONS

Enjoying alcoholic beverages is one way that Pisces temporarily escape the deluge of feelings that often flood them. Yet, as you know, it only provides a temporary reprieve from emotional woes, not a lasting cure. Plus, drowning your sorrows in a sea of Syrah can compromise your liver, leading to reduced energy and immunity. Alcohol is also a diuretic that pulls vital fluid from your body, and therefore, too much is not health-supportive for the water-bound Fish. To make your drinks go further, slowly sip them; this will reduce your alcohol intake (and your bar bill). Enjoy one glass of water for each drink you imbibe to stave off dehydration and the chance of experiencing a hangover headache.

Health-Supporting Foods

There are many nutrient-rich foods from the sea that can give you the energy you need to sustain your giving nature while also helping you feel more grounded, something often challenging for the Fish.

FISH AND SHELLFISH

Not surprisingly, fish and shellfish can play an important role in a healthy Piscean diet. The protein these foods provides gives you long-running energy, while their selenium and zinc help support your immune system. Anti-inflammatory omega-3s—most concentrated in fish such as salmon, sardines, and herring—may promote heart health, help those with mood disorders, and contribute to radiant skin and hair. Seafood can make a quick and easy dinner, with most types taking less than ten minutes to bake, grill, or poach. A can of high-quality salmon or sardines is an easy-to-pack lunchbox addition that you can readily add to a salad or enjoy with a touch of lemon juice and a dash of sea salt.

SEA VEGETABLES

Other great seafoods for Pisces are sea vegetables (also known as seaweed), such as nori, dulse, and kombu. Loaded with minerals—including hard-to-find iodine—sea vegetables make great additions to soups, salads, and, of course, sushi rolls. They also contain phytonutrients known as polysaccharides, which have been found to have anti-inflammatory properties. Add strips of nori, and their spark of phosphorescent color, to a green salad. Dulse flakes (available in prepackaged shakers) make a great on-table condiment. A piece of kombu added when cooking a pot of beans can help guard against legume-related flatulence.

SEA SALT

If you are going to add salt to your meals, consider using sea salt instead of regular table salt. Derived from evaporated seawater rather than land-based halite deposits, mineral-rich sea salt aligns energetically with Pisces' aqueous constitution. Different types of sea salt feature distinctive flavors, from pure and simple to richly oceanic. Experiment with the many varieties of sea salt, as each features a different color, texture, and taste. Some interesting ones include French fleur de sel, pink-colored Hawaiian, and pyramid-shaped Balinese sea salt. Just be careful not to go overboard with your salt intake, which can lead to swelling, especially in those sensitive Piscean feet.

 ## Wellness Therapies

If you feel like escaping from the world, pamper yourself with a wellness treatment, soothing your mind and nurturing your body.

REFLEXOLOGY

Reflexology, a form of bodywork focused almost exclusively on the feet, seems custom-made for Pisces. A reflexology practitioner—often a massage therapist, chiropractor, or podiatrist—reads the feet like a map of the body and applies pressure to the areas corresponding to the body parts that need some extra attention. More than just a simple foot massage, reflexology can give you an overall wellness boost. You can also find reflexology maps online or in books, which will allow you to practice a basic form of this soulful healing technique at home.

HYPNOTHERAPY

Since Pisces are especially open to the thoughts and feelings that reside in their subconscious, hypnotherapy—which facilitates access to this part of the mind—may be an especially effective wellness modality for the Fish. Hypnotherapy is particularly good for reducing chronic pain, counteracting anxiety and insomnia, and alleviating stress-related illnesses. It can also be helpful for releasing addictive behaviors, something with which sensitive Pisces may struggle. Because it's important to feel comfortable and trust your hypnotherapist, take the time to interview several before committing to one. Look for practitioners who are members of professional hypnotherapy societies or associations.

WATSU

Because Pisces are generally at home in the water, Watsu, a form of aquatic bodywork, is well suited to the Fish. During a Watsu session, you float in a pool of warm water while the practitioner gently sways your body. Being suspended in water is not only soothing, but it also allows your body to move in ways that would be impossible on a massage table. It helps relax your muscles, realign your energy, and calm your mind, providing moments of meditative bliss, a cherished haven for spiritually inclined Pisces. You can still find benefit in the therapeutic quality of water even if you are unable to enlist an aquatic bodywork practitioner: spend time floating in a pool or lake, gently supported by a trusted friend.

Relaxation Practices

Taking time to relax, participating in mind-centering activities, and connecting with the deeper parts of yourself can do wonders for a Pisces' sense of well-being.

MEDITATION

Meditation helps calm the churning seas of the mind, body, and spirit. Being still, even for twenty minutes a day, can help you align with the deeper parts of yourself, which is very important for a soul-searching Pisces. In addition to helping you connect with your core being, meditation has many well-documented health benefits: it reduces stress-related illnesses, combats insomnia, and improves heart health. While there are a variety of different techniques to try, mindfulness meditation, breath meditation, and Transcendental Meditation are among the most popular. Don't let time be a barrier that keeps you from meditation: even taking five minutes here and there to center your mind can be beneficial.

SWIMMING

As you might have guessed, swimming is tailor-made for the Fish. It helps you unwind as you fluidly move your body through the water. Swimming provides a cardiovascular workout that's gentle and low impact, perfect for your sensitive temperament. Many colleges and community centers offer swimming courses geared toward a variety of levels. If you don't have access to a pool—or lake, river, or ocean—soaking in a bathtub can do wonders to release tension on both a physical and an emotional level. Lighting candles, playing soft music, and adding fragrant essential oils to the tub can transform a regular bath into a dreamy and relaxing experience.

WALKING

Walking is a gentle form of exercise that allows your Piscean feet to connect to the Earth. Not only will a peaceful promenade calm the mind, but walking also provides the added benefit of stimulating your lymphatic system and strengthening your immunity. Just make sure you wear supportive shoes when out for a walk so that a potentially relaxing experience doesn't transform itself into one spent worrying about your aching feet. As an added Piscean treat, incorporate water into this relaxation practice. For example, after a walk, soak your feet in a footbath infused with sea salt to relax your soles and enliven your spirit.

 # Natural Remedies

Herbs, dietary supplements, and homeopathic remedies are natural ways for Pisces to fortify their physical boundaries.

REISHI MUSHROOMS (*GANODERMA LUCIDUM*)

As Neptune—one of your planetary rulers—is traditionally associated with mushrooms, it makes sense that reishi mushrooms (known as *lingzhi* in Chinese) would be a top pick when it comes to an herbal supplement for the Fish. Used in traditional Chinese medicine for more than two thousand years, *lingzhi* means "herb of spiritual potency," perfect for the soulful Pisces. Reishi is one of the premier adaptogens, a class of herbs that enhance the body's resistance to stress and fatigue, bolstering the immune system. Reishi mushrooms are available in various forms, including capsules, powder, liquid tincture, and tea.

FISH OIL

If you cannot eat omega-3-rich fish—such as salmon, sardines, or herring—several times a week, you may want to consider taking fish oil supplements. The "good" fats contained in fish oil have anti-inflammatory properties and lower cholesterol, lubricate joints, and enhance skin and hair health. People who experience depression are often deficient in this important nutrient. Look for fish oil from manufacturers that use third-party testing to ensure that their products are free of PCBs, heavy metals, and other contaminants. Pisces wanting a vegetarian source of omega-3s should consider flaxseed oil and/or algae supplements.

HOMEOPATHIC PHOSPHORUS

Different homeopathic remedies are associated with distinct psychological constitutions; the one affiliated with homeopathic phosphorus is well matched to the Piscean archetype, that of a person with very fluid boundaries who absorbs the thoughts and feelings of others. It is also a good remedy for nervous tension, insomnia, dizziness, and headaches that are exacerbated by heat and motion. Low-dose phosphorus homeopathics are available in health food stores. Higher-dose forms, which work better as constitutional remedies, are best taken under the guidance of a homeopathic physician. Mint and coffee can counteract the effectiveness of this remedy, so avoid them for several hours before and after taking phosphorus.

 ## Essential Oils

Essential oils provide Pisces with an exquisitely effective way to lift their spirits and connect with their innate psychic and artistic talents.

SANDALWOOD (*SANTALUM ALBUM* AND *SANTALUM SPICATUM*)

Sandalwood oil is derived from the fragrant wood of the sandalwood tree. The smell of sandalwood is said to heighten the ability to make connections between the seen and the unseen worlds, a useful tool to aid in Piscean artistry. It is thought to energize the pineal gland (see page 177)—and by association, psychic gifts. Sandalwood also has other boons: it has aphrodisiac properties and helps quell nervous tension. Dab some sandalwood oil in the center of your forehead to enhance your intuition. Inspire romanticism by misting sandalwood-infused water onto your bed linens. Wear a *japa mala*, a string of Tibetan prayer beads made from sandalwood, so this mystical scent can guide you throughout the day.

MYRRH (*COMMIPHORA MYRRHA*)

Myrrh has been revered for its sacred properties throughout history. It figures prominently in the Bible—being one of the gifts of the magi—as well as in ancient Egyptian texts. Throughout the world, myrrh has been used as incense in holy temples. It has divine skin-care properties as well, great for healing wounds, soothing dry skin, and mollifying heel fissures. When you want a spirit-lifting aroma or an aid to your meditation practice, consider using myrrh in a diffuser to scent a room. Massage your feet with myrrh-scented body lotion to allay dry skin and heal cracked heels.

TEA TREE OIL (*MELALEUCA ALTERNIFOLIA*)

When it comes to warding off infections and buoying the Pisces-ruled immune system, tea tree oil is in a class all its own. Its antiseptic properties are widespread, having antibacterial, antiviral, *and* antifungal activities. Yet its benefits are not limited to the physical: the smell of tea tree oil has mood-elevating properties and inspires feelings of optimism. As tea tree oil can help with athlete's foot, mix some with an unscented body cream and use as needed. If dandruff or dry scalp is a problem, add a few drops to your shampoo.

 # Flower Essences

There's an innate poetry to flower essences that may deeply resonate with a Pisces. (See page 20 for how to use flower essences.)

NICOTIANA (*NICOTIANA ALATA*)

The expansive empathetic nature of Pisces can sometimes make denizens feel like they are drowning in a sea of emotion. In response, many turn to substances (such as tobacco and alcohol) or activities (such as shopping and watching television) through which they can temporarily escape the realities of the world—and the deluge of feelings they can engender. Instead, try Nicotiana flower essence: it can fortify your heart, giving you a floatation aid with which to ride the emotional waves rather than feel submerged by them.

ASPEN (*POPULUS TREMULA*)

Known as the "psychic sponge" of the zodiac, Pisces innately pick up on the thoughts and feelings of others, as well as subtle energies swirling around them. Yet if you absorb these without discernment, it can lead to low-level anxiety and exacerbated worry, which in turn can have you experience heightened fears. Aspen flower essence helps calm the mind, allowing you to better sift through the impressions you receive. This can enhance your powerful perceptive potential, reduce disquietude, and have you feel more confident to navigate the unknown.

PINK YARROW (*ACHILLEA MILLEFOLIUM* VAR. *RUBRA*)

The Fish tends to overidentify with the suffering of others. While your compassionate nature is one of your virtues, if you give away too much of yourself, it can lead to a slow leak in your vital energy. This drain in your energetic resources, combined with your inclination to merge emotionally with others, can make you vulnerable to psychosomatic illness and depressive tendencies. Pink Yarrow flower essence strengthens your fluid personal boundaries, helping you gain objectivity while still maintaining your empathic spirit. This way you can be compassionate without losing your center, or yourself.

 ## Yoga Poses

Pisces often get lost in a sea of their thoughts and feelings, and yoga is a constructive way to do so, as it is a moving meditation that fosters a connection to body, mind, and spirit.

FISH (*MATSYASANA*)

Your namesake pose helps open both the heart chakra—connecting you to feelings of love—and the throat chakra—helping you more fluidly communicate these radiant feelings.

- Lie on your back with your legs outstretched. With your palms on the floor, place your hands under your buttocks. Your forearms should be parallel to the long edge of your yoga mat.

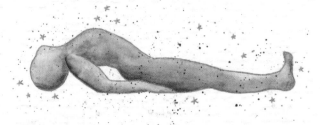

On an inhalation, gently lift your torso. Arching your middle back, tilt your head backward so the crown of your head comes to the floor. Stay in the pose for up to thirty seconds. To come out of the pose, press your forearms into the ground, and on an exhale, gently release your head and lay it on the floor, moving your arms beside your torso.

CHILD (*BALASANA*)

Child pose stretches and massages the feet. Yogis also say that it helps stimulate the third eye, the seat of Piscean psychic abilities.

Kneel on the floor with your knees together and the tops of your feet on the floor. Place your buttocks on your heels, and bend forward until your torso rests on your thighs and your forehead on the floor (or a yoga block). Your arms can be extended out straight in front of you or to your sides with your palms next to your feet. Stay in the pose for as long as needed to feel rejuvenated.

TOE CRUNCH

This descriptively named pose may not have a Sanskrit moniker, but that doesn't detract from the authentic benefits that it can provide. Toe Crunch is one of the best postures around when it comes to circulating energy to your feet.

■ Kneel on the floor with your knees parallel and your toes curled under (so that the bottoms of your feet are at an angle to the floor rather than touching it). Lean forward with your hands gently resting on the floor in front of your knees. You should feel your toes and the balls of your feet opening up. Slowly move toward sitting back on your heels, with your torso vertical (or until the point where it gets uncomfortable). Stay in the pose for up to one minute with mini-rest breaks as needed.

Inspiring Sleep

Your empathetic nature may have you taking on more than your fair share of others' emotions during the day. This may leave you swimming in a reservoir of feelings—whether of abundant joy, sorrow, or anxiousness—when night falls, which can keep you from easily shifting into sleep. To embrace greater inner peace, acknowledge both the worries and the beauties of the day, and then give yourself permission to let them go, as you let go into the land of Nod.

stellar life stages

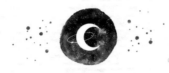

STELLAR LIFE STAGES THROUGH THE AGES

As you saw in Part I, your personal astrology chart can be a periscope that provides you with stellar guidance to foster your well-being. Even just knowing your Sun sign—and that of your Moon and Ascendant signs (see pages 12–14)—can help you optimize your health and vitality.

Yet, the wellness-inspiring awareness that your personal planetary profile yields extends beyond that, which is the focus of Part II. Here you'll discover a way to navigate through different periods of your life—from your twenties to your eighties—with the greater self-knowledge that astrology grants. I offer you a simplified approach to a complex astrological realm to arm you with insights to embrace more clarity and confidence.

Self-Knowledge Throughout Life

In addition to the unique understanding we can gain about our self-care needs by becoming familiar with our birth chart, astrology also offers us the ability to understand the opportunities and challenges that different periods in our life may contain. Knowing this—what we're being called to learn and the possible stressors we may need to navigate—allows us the foresight to identify ways we can best support ourselves during different stages of life.

How our life unfolds is, of course, unique to all of us, and with the help of your birth chart, an astrologer can help you better understand your personal life map. Birth charts provide you with what can be considered as a customized weather report, a snapshot into

Spanning Time

Stellar Life Stages occur when a planet in the sky makes a connection to where it was in your birth chart. The reason that these occur at a pretty similar age for each of us is because every planet has a consistent orbital period. For example, since it takes Jupiter twelve years to travel around the Sun, everyone has their Jupiter Return (see pages 194–195)—when the planet resides in the same location in the sky it was when they were born—every dozen or so years. And while there is a precise moment that it revisits that celestial spot, Stellar Life Stages, as you'll see, are not one-day events, but are rather experienced over a year or two. That's because a planet's astrological invitation can be felt for some time before and after the actual astronomical event occurs.

what the different climates of your life may feel like at different times. Astrologers determine this timing map using techniques such as transits (looking at the relationship between where the planets currently are and where they were when you were born) and progressions (observing how your chart evolves throughout time).

While we each have our own individual "climate report"—since we each have a unique star chart—there are some planetary cycles we all experience at the same time as our peers. Knowing about these—which I call Stellar Life Stages—can help you better chart the cycles of your life, giving you further understanding of the challenges and opportunities that different moments yield. Knowing what Stellar Life Stage you may be currently moving through, or are approaching, gives you a compass that can help you more consciously navigate the situations you may face. And, it can also help you design self-care strategies that will best support your well-being as your life evolves.

In the following sections, you will learn about the Stellar Life Stages associated with six planets and celestial bodies. You'll see the age range when each occurs and you'll discover the lessons that each passage may be highlighting; since knowledge is power, this information will help you stave off stress as well as assist you in making more conscious decisions, both inherent components of well-being. Each Stellar Life Stage also includes a wellness strategy, a way to orient your self-care throughout this time, and flower essences that can help you flourish. (See page 20 for how to use flower essences.) Additionally, you'll find several Stellar Reflections journaling prompts you can use to dig deeper into the awareness that each period beckons.

To briefly illustrate this concept, let's consider the Saturn Return (see pages 196–197), which probably the most well-known Stellar Life Stage. Given that it takes the multiringed planet about twenty-nine years to complete one revolution, everyone will move through this Stellar Life Stage when they are around thirty, and then again when they are shy of sixty and ninety. Knowing that this is a time when you are poised to embrace Saturnian lessons—such as the wisdom of aging, the recognition of limits, the importance of strong foundations, and the acknowledgment of your inner authority—will allow you to perceive events that manifest during these years using this lens of awareness. Saturn-inspired self-care approaches that are steeped in tradition can help you strengthen your physical structure and let you feel more in charge during this time.

So that you can have an overview of these Stellar Life Stages and how they may weave through the tapestry of your life, on page 193 you'll find a chart called Stellar Life Stages Through the Ages. There you can look to see, based upon your age, which stage you may be passing through, or may have just experienced, or will move through shortly. You'll see that these stages unfold in several ways. At some points in our life we experience only one Stellar Life Stage; while during other times in our life, one stage will flow into another; and at other moments in our life, we may experience two stages simultaneously.

Returns, Squares, and Oppositions

Stellar Life Stages are determined based upon each planet's orbital pathway and how long it takes it to complete either a full—or partial—cycle around the Sun. Here's a quick primer on some astrological terms to help you better understand them.

Return: When a planet arrives back at the same place in the zodiac it occupied when you were born, the planet is said to be experiencing a return.

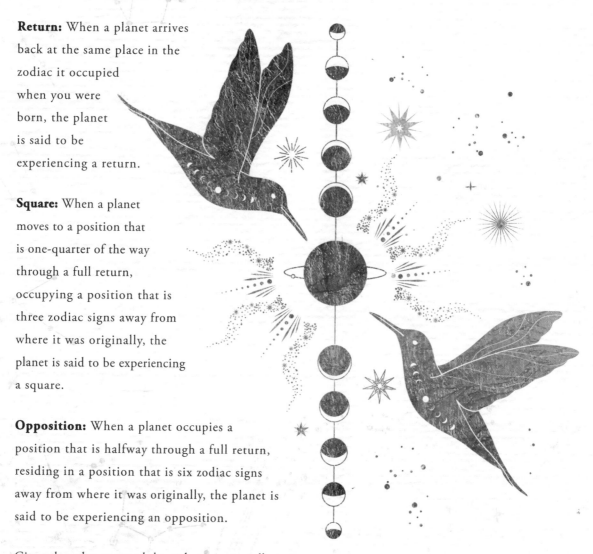

Square: When a planet moves to a position that is one-quarter of the way through a full return, occupying a position that is three zodiac signs away from where it was originally, the planet is said to be experiencing a square.

Opposition: When a planet occupies a position that is halfway through a full return, residing in a position that is six zodiac signs away from where it was originally, the planet is said to be experiencing an opposition.

Given that planets travel through some constellations more quickly than others, a planetary square and opposition don't necessarily equate to it spending one-quarter or one-half, respectively, of the entire time of its orbit. For example, you'll notice that for those who are currently having their Pluto Square, it's occurring when they are 40–42, which is less than a fourth of this dwarf planet's 248-year orbit.

Stellar Life Stages Through the Ages

YOUR TWENTIES

YOUR THIRTIES

YOUR FORTIES

YOUR FIFTIES

YOUR SIXTIES

YOUR SEVENTIES

YOUR EIGHTIES

* Owing to Pluto's orbit and it spending varying amounts of time in each zodiac sign, the age at which different generations experience their Pluto Square differs. It's those who were born between 1981 to 1986 who will experience

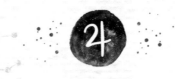

JUPITER RETURN

Occurs when Jupiter—the planet that reflects understanding, expansion, and faith—returns to the realm of the sky it occupied when you were born. Jupiter's orbit around the Sun takes approximately 12 years.

You'll experience your **Jupiter Return** when you are:

- 23–24 years old
- 35–36 years old
- 47–48 years old
- 59–60 years old
- 71–72 years old
- 82–83 years old

About every twelve years, we experience a Jupiter Return, a time that offers us an opportunity to set our sights upon a new horizon. When we're moving through this Stellar Life Stage, we sense that a chapter is ending and that we are about to embark upon another stage of growth. During this period, we hear the call of our Higher Self; if we listen to the wisdom that resides within us, we can become quite clear as to the life direction we want to pursue. And while it's a time when opportunity regularly knocks, it's important that we be discerning and not take every offer available, or else we may find ourselves frittering away our resources. Have your choices be aligned with intentionality, benevolence, and generosity, so that when Jupiter's encouragement arrives it can propel you toward growth that promotes both you and the social good. At the same time, watch that this period's propensity for optimism and expansion doesn't have you excelling at being excessive, extravagant, or careless.

WELLNESS STRATEGY: BE EXPLORATORY

Given that the Jupiter Return is a time for learning as well as broadening your vistas, explore wellness approaches from other cultures: for example, research healing herbs from South America, nutrient-rich foods from Asia, and relaxation strategies from Scandinavian countries. As you embrace a forward-looking bent, and take advantage of an urge to define new goals, creating vision boards can help you set your sights upon what you want to discover and manifest. Whether it's training for a half-marathon, meditating daily for twenty minutes, limiting alcohol to the weekends, or some other aim, envisioning and working toward your objective will yield positive reward. While this is a time of optimism and enjoyment, be attuned to what you're eating so that the affinity for growth you experience doesn't manifest in your waistline. Flower essences to explore include Angelica, Shasta Daisy, and Vervain.

STELLAR REFLECTIONS

Who is my role model when it comes to living life with positivity and enthusiasm?

....

....

....

What new goals do I want to set?

....

....

....

What am I inspired to learn?

....

....

....

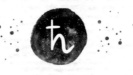

SATURN RETURN

Occurs when Saturn—the planet that reflects limits, time, and responsibility—returns to the realm of the sky it occupied when you were born. Saturn's orbit around the Sun takes approximately 29.5 years.

You'll experience your **Saturn Return** when you are:

- 29–30 years old
- 58–59 years old
- 87–88 years old

The Saturn Return is a period when time becomes a great teacher, and when we make a deeper commitment to how we truly want to author our life. During this Stellar Life Stage we may find ourselves at a crossroads, needing to untangle from choices previously made that we've come to realize mirror the preferences of others rather than those of our true self. And with this, we may find ourselves dealing with crisis, conflicts, or the big life decisions for which the Saturn Return is often associated. As we embrace the power to say no, we continue to see how it helps us act in concert with what we truly know is right for us. We move from feeling like we are just executing other people's plans to a sense that we are a responsible architect of our own life, building beautiful things in which we truly believe. The first Saturn Return is thought to be a rite of passage into adulthood when we more confidently invoke the authority within us; the second is a time when we pare down to knowing more clearly what is essential to how we want to live our lives; the third is when we even more deeply stand in the wisdom we have honed.

WELLNESS STRATEGY: BE DISCIPLINED

One of the lessons of the Saturn Return is to own our authority and more clearly perceive our capacity for conscious commitment. With this, we can discover the power inherent in discipline and setting limits. To this aim, it's a period when you can foster your well-being by dedicating yourself to new thoughtful habits. For example, if you find that you eat too many sweets or drink too many libations, you can embrace a "less is more" strategy and discover your willpower for restraint. Because an appreciation for limits and rule setting flourishes during this time, you may find that creating new regimens that strengthen your body and mind can really pay off. Exercise routines that follow a consistent or rigorous protocol—such as Pilates or Ashtanga yoga—may become more interesting. Dedicating yourself to a practice that takes commitment and is steeped in tradition—for example, meditation or martial arts—can also yield great benefits. Flower essences to explore include Gentian, Walnut, and Wild Oat.

STELLAR REFLECTIONS

What life goals truly feel aligned with who I am?

....

....

....

How can I connect more deeply to the authority within me?

....

....

....

What is it that I truly stand for?

....

....

....

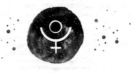

PLUTO SQUARE

Occurs when Pluto—the planet that reflects survival instincts, power, and transformation—occupies a realm of the sky that is one-quarter of the way through its full zodiacal cycle. Pluto's orbit around the Sun takes approximately 248 years.

You'll experience your **Pluto Square** when you are:

- 40–42 years old (this timing of this Stellar Life Stage varies more than others; see the bottom of page 193 for more details)

The Pluto Square marks a time of great intensity in our lives, one in which we find ourselves diving deep below the surface of superficiality to unearth meaning that exists when we tap into the darkness. During this intense Stellar Life Stage in which everything seems to have more significance, even decisions about the most trivial of subjects may take on a life-or-death urgency. We sense the importance of facing our fears and realize we can't go on clinging to situations that leave us disempowered. We burrow into a deep well of faith that can help us release that which has reached its expiration date—whether belief systems, relationships, habits, or the like—even if we don't yet know what will arise in its place. We experience a dismantling that leads to rebuilding from the roots. And like the mythological phoenix, we emerge transformed, regenerated with an indelible capacity for living life with more depth and breadth.

WELLNESS STRATEGY: GO DEEP

During the Pluto Square we learn the necessity of surrender and releasing things that no longer embody vitality and don't truly serve the fullness of who we are. As such, doing activities that involve letting go may help support our well-being. These can include such routines as exfoliating your skin, doing detox fasts, or eliminating suspected allergens from your diet. It can also involve mundane pursuits such as regularly deep cleaning your closets or weeding the garden. Because this is a Stellar Life Stage when we may feel more connected to the cycles of life, contemplating end-of-life matters—whether through conversations with friends and family or reading about different spiritual perspectives— may feel aligned. Also, because this marks a period in which we're looking at matters often shrouded from sight—including those in our subconscious—you may find working with a therapist to be a powerful wellness pursuit. Flower essences to explore include Cherry Plum, Mustard, and Sagebrush.

STELLAR REFLECTIONS

What is my biggest fear?

....

....

....

What beliefs or habits do I want to release?

....

....

....

How can I tap into a deeper reservoir of trust?

....

....

....

....

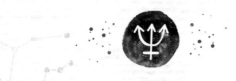

NEPTUNE SQUARE

Occurs when Neptune—the planet that represents spirituality, transcendence, and the imagination—occupies a realm of the sky that is one-quarter of the way through its full zodiacal cycle. Neptune's orbit around the Sun takes approximately 165 years.

You'll experience your **Neptune Square** when you are:

- 40–42 years old

Neptune is associated with the intrinsic qualities of water; consequently, this Stellar Life Stage is often marked by a feeling of dissolution. It may be accompanied by a sense that the structures that we thought to be solid—such as our goals, beliefs, or even the ways we organize our days—appear as if they are losing form to be reformed. It may also be a time of disillusion, in which we may find ourselves exceptionally disappointed if things don't meet our ideals. The Neptune Square may feel like a hazy time, in which our go-to approaches suddenly feel as though they leave us zapped, our energy dissipated, or our brains a bit foggy. Invariably, though, all of this can lead us on a journey in which we further appreciate the reward of going with the flow, trusting our intuition, accessing our compassion, and showering ourselves with love. It's a period when we may find ourselves mourning the dreams that we had for our life. And yet through this process, in which we may feel flooded with feelings, we reconnect to the soul of what it was that originally inspired us; by doing so, we find ourselves reinspired and ready to embark upon a new stream of life.

WELLNESS STRATEGY: BE NUMINOUS

During the Neptune Square, we feel connected to the subtle and diffuse; echoing this, turning to contemplative and reflective practices may provide you with a trusted compass to more confidently sail through this time. For example, commit to a meditation practice, read spiritual texts, or hone your intuition through working with tarot cards. Pay attention to your dreams, honoring them for the whispers of wisdom that they bring. And, given Neptune's association with the aquatic, turn to the healing power of water—whether that's by soaking in the tub, doing footbaths, or listening to seascape sounds. Because this is a period in which we get a clearer lens into our escape patterns, you may find that you have extra insight and stamina to kick a habit to which you've been clinging—whether smoking, drinking too much, excessive TV bingeing, or something else. Flower essences to explore include Clematis, Pink Yarrow, and Star Tulip.

STELLAR REFLECTIONS

How can I further trust my intuition to direct me toward the right path?

....

....

....

How does it feel when I'm going with the flow?

....

....

....

How can I further attend to my spiritual life?

....

....

....

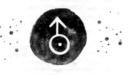

URANUS OPPOSITION

Occurs when Uranus—the planet that reflects innovation, sudden revelations, and rebellions—occupies a realm of the sky that is one-half of the way through its full zodiacal cycle. Uranus's orbit around the Sun takes approximately 84 years. **Note:** *Although the Uranus Square and Uranus Return are distinct from the Uranus Opposition, they all feature similar invitations.*

You'll experience your **Uranus Opposition** when you are:

- 43–45 years old*

You'll experience your **Uranus Square** when you are:

- 20–22 years old and 63–65 years old

You'll experience your **Uranus Return** when you are:

- 83–84 years old

When Uranus in the sky connects to Uranus in your chart, it often coincides with a shake-up, a time when you feel called to shake off the *would-of's* and *should-of's* that have left you feeling overly constrained. It's a Stellar Life Stage filled with surprises, not the least of which is our being surprised at ourselves; it's as if, all of a sudden, we see more clearly who we are, and who we are not. We also get frequent glimpses into whether the way we crafted our life is—or isn't—allowing us to truly express our individual nature. Breaking and remaking patterns, giving ourselves permission to claim our independent spirit, itching to feel more youthful, and experimenting with innovative solutions are just some of the hallmarks of this midlife transition moment. We uncover a clarity of what we

* *Those born before 1970 had their Uranus Opposition a year or two before this age range.*

want alongside the courageous resolve to be unapologetically authentic. And, as we find ourselves leaning toward disruption as a way out of ennui, we see that going against things can offer a pathway that allows us to go *for* what we truly cherish.

WELLNESS STRATEGY: BE INNOVATIVE

Be experimental with your wellness regimen. Try a form of exercise or a relaxation practice you've yet to investigate; you may just surprise yourself with how much you like it. And even if not, the experience of breaking out of routines will leave you feeling more liberated. Speaking of routines, shaking up the order of your daily ones will help you see things through a new lens. Because Uranus is associated with the innovative, complementary, and alternative approaches to healing may pique your curiosity even more than usual; and since this planet also rules the electric, it may be therapies that involve your bio-energetic system that become especially intriguing. For example, give acupuncture a whirl (see page 167), or learn more about gem elixirs. Flower essences to explore include Aspen, Corn, and Yarrow.

STELLAR REFLECTIONS

What unclaimed part of myself do I now want to claim?

How can I infuse my life with a sense of youthfulness?

How can I feel more free?

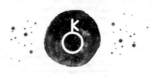

CHIRON RETURN

Occurs when Chiron returns to the same place in the sky it was when you were born. Discovered in 1977, Chiron is a celestial body that orbits between Saturn and Uranus. It has come to be associated with the archetype of the "wounded healer." Chiron's orbit around the Sun takes approximately 50 years.

You'll experience your **Chiron Return** when you are:

- 49–50 years old

As we transition from our forties to our fifties, it often seems that we reach a significant evolutionary point. We become even more conscious of the wounds we carry, and we realize that an essential choice beckons: we can continue to feel dissipated by our hurts or sense of inadequacy, or we can embrace our imperfections and channel them for the higher good. In doing the latter, we galvanize the gifts we have to help others and discover how accepting ourselves is a powerful healing balm. We get more clarity on the root of our suffering and how our judgment and desire for perfection have allowed us to hold on to our wounds, using them to rewound ourselves. Ideally, with this insight, we can rewind and stop the cycle of suffering to embrace ourselves with compassion and transform our handicaps into healing treasures we can offer the world.

WELLNESS STRATEGY: WELCOME HEALING

Seek out self-care approaches that can make you more aware about the heart of your sorrows. Whether it's counseling, hypnosis, or eye movement desensitization and reprocessing (EMDR), explore therapies that can lead you to the roots of your pain and ameliorate the bruises you carry. Given that the mythic Chiron was a wise centaur esteemed for his knowledge of medicine and music, consider taking up an instrument or engaging in wellness practices that involve sound (see page 41). Because the root of Chiron's name (*cheir*) means "hand," explore chiropractic or hands-on healing for the benefits they may offer. Additionally, share insights you've gained about your favorite realms of self-care with others to inspire their path of well-being. Flower essences to explore include Pine, Self-Heal, and Star of Bethlehem.

STELLAR REFLECTIONS

What are my unique healing gifts?

....
....
....
....

What self-limiting stories do I want to release?

....
....
....
....

How can my firsthand experience of sorrow help me help others?

....
....
....
....

PART III:

the moons

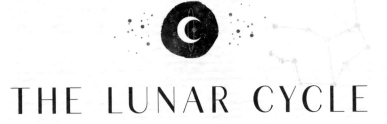

THE LUNAR CYCLE

The Moon has forever pulled on the tides of our imagination. A source of both wonder and worship, it's been revered by cultures the world over, memorialized in legends, myths, and artwork. It reminds us of how in change we find constancy. It's a guiding light and chaperone in the dark night, seen as both beacon and bellwether.

It's no surprise, then, that the Moon plays a starring role in astrology. It governs emotions, maternal inclinations, habitual patterns, and the expression of nurturance. As we saw on page 13, our Moon sign can give us cosmic cues as to which wellness approaches we may find nourishing. Additionally, as it moves more quickly than other planets (a lunar cycle—the time from one New Moon to the next—is 29.5 days), it is also a key feature of numerous astrological timing techniques. And, of course, the shifting appearance of the Moon during the monthly lunar cycle helps us align with a sense of natural rhythm, which can have us feeling connected to both ourselves and the world around us. Let's explore how keying in to the Moon's cycle—notably turning to the wisdom of the New and Full Moons—can serve as a way to understand and sequence a stellar self-care approach.

The Moon's Cycle

The monthly lunar cycle begins with a New Moon. During this lunation, when the Moon resides between the Earth and the Sun, its radiant side is obscured from our view. And while it appears to be absent of any luminosity, the New Moon has traditionally been seen as a time that is filled with great promise, as it ushers in new beginnings. On the New Moon, as well as a few days after, we reconnect to a desire for new growth, setting intentions and planting seeds for what we want to flourish.

The period between a New Moon and Full Moon, as we see more and more of the Moon glowing in light, is referred to as its waxing phase. This two-week period is thought to be the best time to initiate projects that you'd like to develop and expand. For example, if you want to commit to learning a new skill, beginning an exercise regimen, or pursuing a long-term wellness goal, it's thought that doing so during the waxing phase is ideal.

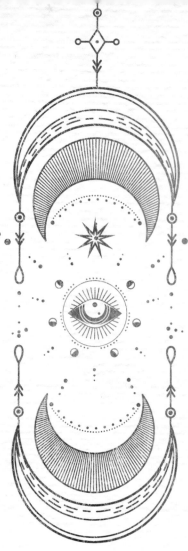

The Full Moon lighting up the sky accords with the Earth residing between the two luminaries (the Sun and Moon), allowing us to see the face of the Moon fully illuminated by the Sun's rays. Emotions may strongly ebb and flow on the days surrounding the Full Moon, a time when awareness is heightened, we recognize new truths and we find ourselves infused with more clarity.

After the Full Moon, darkness begins to take the place of light. The period in which radiance recedes from the face of the Moon, and we move again towards a New Moon, is called the waning phase. Activities that rely upon reduction for achieving success are thought to do well when initiated during this two-week period. Examples of such self-care undertakings include exfoliating your skin, doing a mini-fast, and trimming your hair.

The days just before the New Moon, when the little light there is continues to diminish, is the lunar phase known as the Balsamic Moon. It's a time when we're encouraged to be reflective, turning inward to find awareness that can brighten our path. Dreamwork, meditation, and journaling are wonderful self-care activities to do during this time.

Being in concert with the rhythms of the lunar cycle can help us feel more aligned. Whether it's honoring beginnings at the New Moon or perceiving fruition at the Full Moon, doing activities that extol expansion during the waxing phase, or those that revere restriction during the waning phase, there's a feeling of ease that arises when we're in tune with the Moon.

Yet, how a New Moon or a Full Moon may help us to understand ways in which we can sequence our self-care strategies extends beyond this. On the following pages, you'll learn about the opportunities and challenges that each of the different New and Full Moons hold. To help you tap into their invitation for healing, you'll also find affirmations, self-care rituals, and Stellar Reflection journaling prompts that are in alignment with each. These will help you invite in awareness while also side-stepping stress, using the Moon as a guiding light that can chaperone you on your journey for optimal well-being.

While calendars and almanacs usually include the dates of New and Full Moons (as well as First and Last Quarter Moons), they often don't include their zodiac positions. To find a resource for this information, see page 252.

Eclipses

Every year, between four and seven eclipses grace the sky. Solar eclipses accord with New Moons while lunar eclipses correspond with Full Moons. These celestial events are renowned for occurring in sync with life-changing events or reflections. Given that this often accords with excitement, stress, and/or heightened energy, it's important to pay special attention to your body and mind during eclipse season. Carve out extra time for relaxation practices, boost your diet's nutrient richness, and make sure you're getting adequate sleep: these can bolster your strength and resilience so that you navigate this transformational time with more confidence and consciousness.

NEW MOONS

When a New Moon occurs, the Sun and Moon occupy the same zodiac sign. Given there are twelve signs (see page 16), there are actually a dozen different New Moons that occur every year, with each one having a different astrological ambience. With a New Moon being a time of beginnings, we often find that the realm of life being sparked for expansion is related to the sign that is being highlighted. For example, during an Aries New Moon, everyone—regardless of their astrology profile—may find themselves galvanized with energy, wanting to act quickly at the behest of fresh pursuits. Compare that with a Libra New Moon, when we're tuned into recalibrating relationship dynamics so that our partnerships can bring us more pleasure. By zeroing in on the characteristics of the sign that's highlighted during the New Moon, you become aware of the opportunities for learning that the moment may offer. On the following pages you will find insights that will help you amplify your self-care for each New Moon.

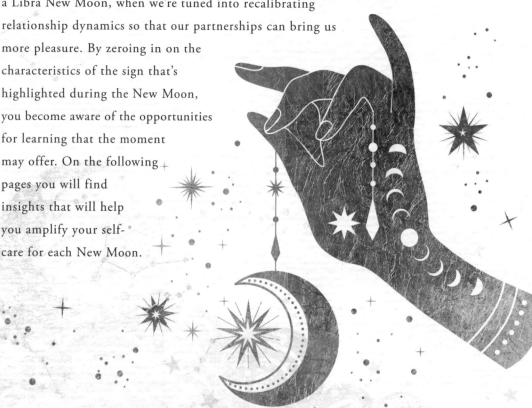

Aries New Moon

THE OPPORTUNITIES

- Finding the courage to begin something you've been avoiding.
- Discovering a cause for which you want to fight.

THE CHALLENGES

- Moving fast could lead to minor accidents or mishaps.
- A now-or-never orientation catalyzes a rash of impatience, irritation, and anger.

AFFIRMATIONS

- I lay claim to my desires.
- I am brave.
- I am energized.
- The present moment informs me deeply.

SELF-CARE RITUALS

- Exercise outdoors.
- Add some spice to your meals.

STELLAR REFLECTIONS

What do I want to champion?

....

....

What incites my passion?

....

....

What can help me be more patient?

....

....

Taurus New Moon

THE OPPORTUNITIES

- Surveying habits to see which are truly supportive.
- Looking to nature for guidance and grounding.

THE CHALLENGES

- A swell of stubbornness limits adaptability.
- Focusing too much on the mundane without looking under the surface.

AFFIRMATIONS

- My senses delight and inform me.
- Being practical yields great possibilities.
- The Earth supports and nurtures me.
- I am safe.

SELF-CARE RITUALS

- Listen to music.
- Buy yourself flowers.

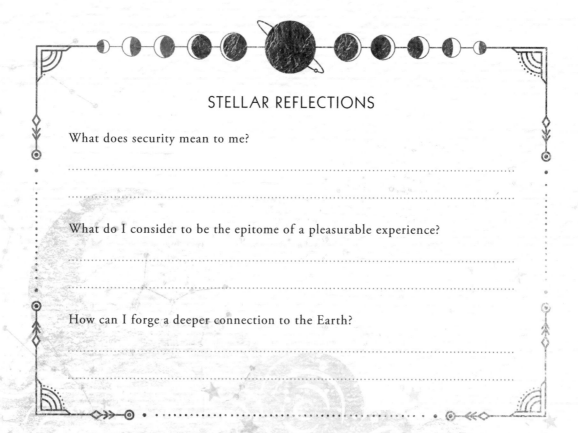

STELLAR REFLECTIONS

What does security mean to me?

....

....

What do I consider to be the epitome of a pleasurable experience?

....

....

How can I forge a deeper connection to the Earth?

....

....

Gemini New Moon

THE OPPORTUNITIES

- Discovering solutions through conversations.
- Having a greater ability to be flexible and versatile.

THE CHALLENGES

- Limited attention span and difficulty concentrating.
- With so much information to process, nervous energy abounds.

AFFIRMATIONS

- My mind is bright.
- Knowledge is power.
- I am flexible.
- I speak with confidence and clarity.

SELF-CARE RITUALS

- Begin a new magazine or book.
- Call up a friend.

STELLAR REFLECTIONS

What am I really curious about right now?

....

....

When my mind feels scattered, what are my go-to practices to center myself?

....

....

What's my unique learning style?

....

....

Cancer New Moon

THE OPPORTUNITIES

- Honoring your emotions and letting them guide you.
- Exploring who and what has you feeling more at home in the world.

THE CHALLENGES

- An emphasis on the emotional may obscure the rational.
- A tendency to move in a slow and indirect manner may yield frustrations.

AFFIRMATIONS

- I trust my emotions.
- I know how to take care of myself.
- I feel protected.
- I am nourished.

SELF-CARE RITUALS

- Prepare a home-cooked meal.
- Reach out to a relative.

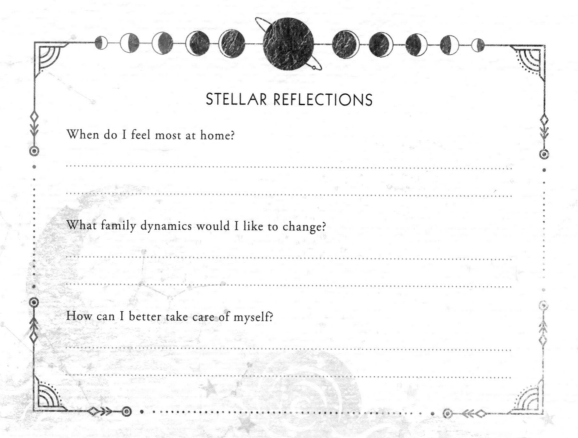

STELLAR REFLECTIONS

When do I feel most at home?

....

....

What family dynamics would I like to change?

....

....

How can I better take care of myself?

....

Leo New Moon

THE OPPORTUNITIES

- Becoming more generous in how you express your love.
- Being creative and expressing your unique self.

THE CHALLENGES

- People may be prickly, notably if their pride is wounded.
- A fear of embarrassment may keep you from sharing your talents.

AFFIRMATIONS

- My heart is a stream of love.
- Being generous makes my life richer.
- I am bold.
- I feel royal.

SELF-CARE RITUALS

- Do an artistic project.
- Spend time with a child.

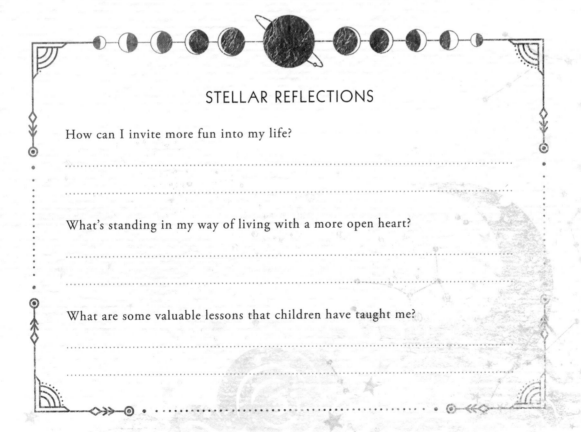

STELLAR REFLECTIONS

How can I invite more fun into my life?

....

....

What's standing in my way of living with a more open heart?

....

....

What are some valuable lessons that children have taught me?

....

....

Virgo New Moon

THE OPPORTUNITIES

- Paying attention to the details leads to a solution.

- Finding ways to be of service to others.

THE CHALLENGES

- A penchant for perfection can cause heightened criticality.

- Excess worry and anxiety can occur when things appear out of order.

AFFIRMATIONS

- I am of service.

- I am enough.

- I see the parts and I see the whole.

- Perfection is an illusion.

SELF-CARE RITUALS

- Organize your files or kitchen cabinets.

- Do a craft project.

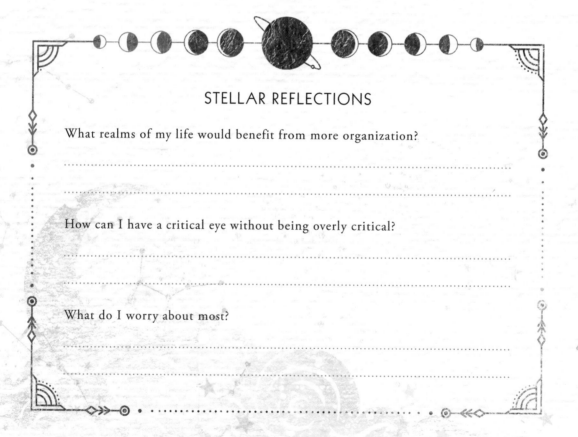

STELLAR REFLECTIONS

What realms of my life would benefit from more organization?

....

....

How can I have a critical eye without being overly critical?

....

....

What do I worry about most?

....

....

Libra New Moon

THE OPPORTUNITIES

- Discovering how alliances make your life more enjoyable.
- Exploring pathways that create equitable outcomes.

THE CHALLENGES

- Compromising your needs in an attempt to keep the peace.
- An aversion to making a wrong choice could lead to procrastination.

AFFIRMATIONS

- Equality is important to me.
- I trust my choices.
- I am a good ally.
- I am beauty.

SELF-CARE RITUALS

- Plan a social gathering.
- Read poetry.

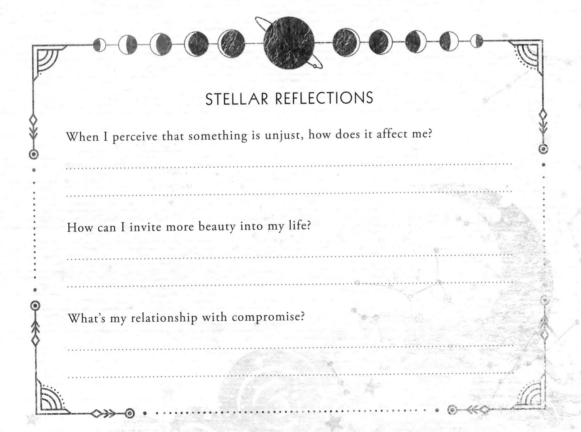

STELLAR REFLECTIONS

When I perceive that something is unjust, how does it affect me?

....

....

How can I invite more beauty into my life?

....

....

What's my relationship with compromise?

....

....

Scorpio New Moon

THE OPPORTUNITIES

- Connecting to an unwavering commitment.
- Mining your emotions to better understand what you are feeling.

THE CHALLENGES

- An all-or-nothing orientation that leaves no middle ground.
- Truth may be veiled with people assuming a more secretive stance.

AFFIRMATIONS

- Treasures reside under the surface.
- My desires run deep.
- The dark is illuminating.
- I trust my emotions.

SELF-CARE RITUALS

- Deep clean your closets.
- Practice intermittent fasting.

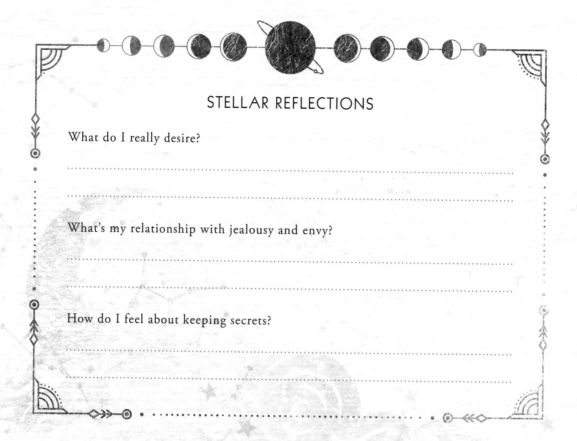

STELLAR REFLECTIONS

What do I really desire?

....

....

What's my relationship with jealousy and envy?

....

....

How do I feel about keeping secrets?

....

Sagittarius New Moon

THE OPPORTUNITIES

- Envisioning what you'd like your future to look like.
- Exploring philosophical or spiritual wisdom.

THE CHALLENGES

- Overenthusiasm can lead to exhaustion.
- An overly zealous perspective may rub others the wrong way.

AFFIRMATIONS

- I give myself permission to aim high.
- I am wise.
- My vision is clear.
- I have faith.

SELF-CARE RITUALS

- Create a vision board.
- Read a travel magazine.

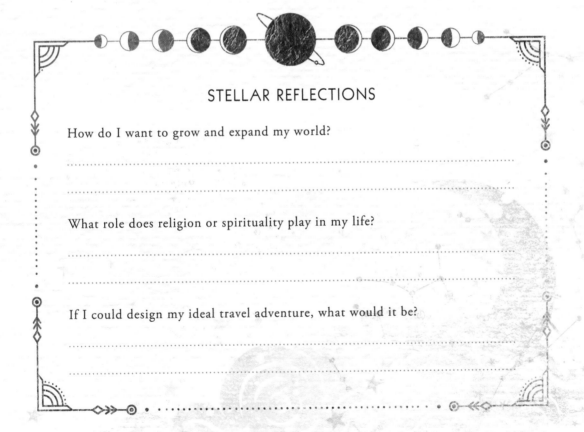

STELLAR REFLECTIONS

How do I want to grow and expand my world?

....

....

What role does religion or spirituality play in my life?

....

....

If I could design my ideal travel adventure, what would it be?

....

....

Capricorn New Moon

THE OPPORTUNITIES

- Defining an achievement toward which you'd like to work.

- Appreciating how creating solid foundations builds lasting structures.

THE CHALLENGES

- An emphasis on being dutiful may create a somber environment.

- Hard work may lead to burnout.

AFFIRMATIONS

- I am responsible.

- Success is within my reach.

- Loyalty is an asset.

- I have endurance.

SELF-CARE RITUALS

- Work on a financial budget.

- Do some stretching exercises.

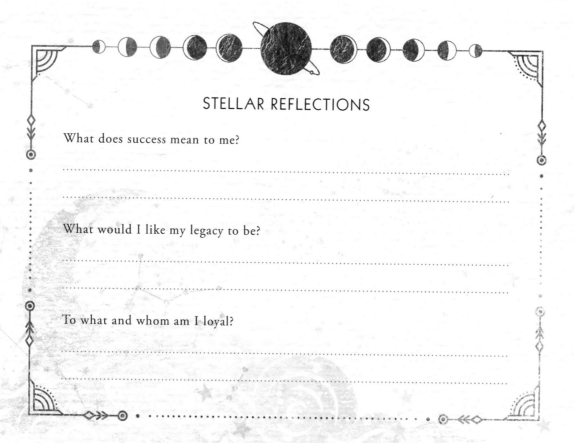

STELLAR REFLECTIONS

What does success mean to me?

....

....

What would I like my legacy to be?

....

....

To what and whom am I loyal?

....

....

Aquarius New Moon

THE OPPORTUNITIES

- Exploring how a new technology offers unique solutions.
- Investigating innovative and alternative approaches to well-being.

THE CHALLENGES

- An emphasis on the rational that doesn't consider the emotional.
- Sacrificing your personal needs to support those of a group.

AFFIRMATIONS

- I am a citizen of the world.
- Collectives have power.
- I can sense subtle energies.
- I can help make a difference.

SELF-CARE RITUALS

- Meditate with crystals.
- Do a community project.

STELLAR REFLECTIONS

What three things can I do to make the world a better place?

....

....

Which tech devices do I most rely upon?

....

....

Which communities or groups align with my vision and values?

....

....

Pisces New Moon

THE OPPORTUNITIES

- Connecting to a more soulful way of perceiving life.
- Being more empathetic and compassionate.

THE CHALLENGES

- An oversensitivity to others can lead to blurred boundaries.
- Difficulty in discerning what's truly real from what you want to be real.

AFFIRMATIONS

- Dreams can come true.
- We are all connected.
- I am love.
- I am loved.

SELF-CARE RITUALS

- Take a bath.
- Make art.

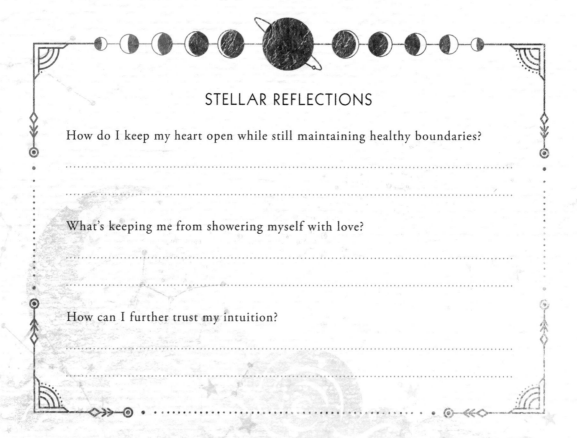

STELLAR REFLECTIONS

How do I keep my heart open while still maintaining healthy boundaries?

What's keeping me from showering myself with love?

How can I further trust my intuition?

FULL MOONS

Just as there are twelve different New Moons annually, there are also a dozen distinct Full Moons, each taking place when the Sun is in a different zodiac sign. Since a Full Moon occurs when the Sun and Moon are on opposite sides of the Earth (see page 208), this lunation features the luminaries that are opposite each other in the zodiac. Therefore, each Full Moon invites us to synthesize needs that seem to run counter to each other, and yet by doing so we can expand our capacity for conscious living. Each one offers us unique experiences and lessons. For example, during the Cancer Full Moon—featuring the Sun in responsible Capricorn and the Moon in nurturing Cancer—we may find ourselves pulled between attending to the demands of our career while we also strive to balance family responsibilities. Compare this to the invitation of the Pisces Full Moon; with the Sun in fastidious Virgo and the Moon in dreamy Pisces, it's a time when we need to hone the focus of our rational mind but not at the expense of the beauty that can emerge when we tap into our intuition and imagination.

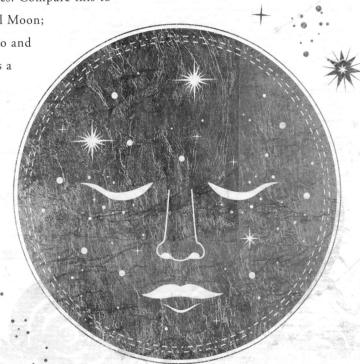

On the following pages you will find insights that will help you elevate your well-being for each Full Moon.

Aries Full Moon

THE OPPORTUNITIES

- Discovering the will to go the extra distance for someone.
- Being a champion for beauty, justice, and peace.

THE CHALLENGES

- Having little patience when perceiving that something is unfair.
- Sensing a divide between what's best for you and what's best for a relationship.

AFFIRMATIONS

- I fight for justice.
- My will is strong.
- I deserve pleasure.
- I am a good friend.

SELF-CARE RITUALS

- Give yourself a facial.
- Exercise with a friend.

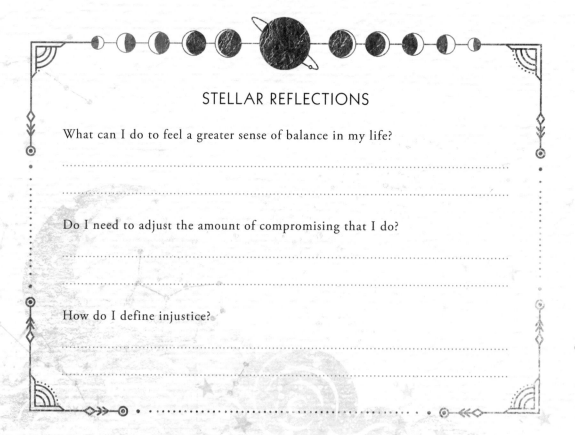

STELLAR REFLECTIONS

What can I do to feel a greater sense of balance in my life?

....

....

Do I need to adjust the amount of compromising that I do?

....

....

How do I define injustice?

....

....

Taurus Full Moon

THE OPPORTUNITIES

- Feeling nourished by sensual experiences.
- Seeing how practical solutions yield transformative outcomes.

THE CHALLENGES

- Lack of flexibility may restrict options.
- Resistance to staying with powerful emotions.

AFFIRMATIONS

- I am safe and secure.
- I can manifest.
- My sensuality nurtures me.
- My beauty runs deep.

SELF-CARE RITUALS

- Do a mud mask.
- Exfoliate your skin.

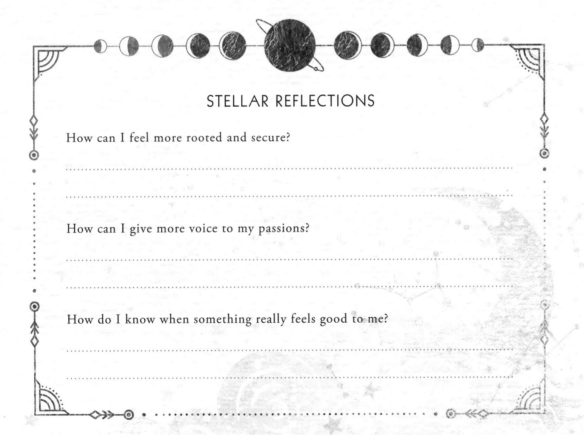

STELLAR REFLECTIONS

How can I feel more rooted and secure?

....

....

How can I give more voice to my passions?

....

....

How do I know when something really feels good to me?

....

....

Gemini Full Moon

THE OPPORTUNITIES

- Gathering more data to bolster your message.
- Discovering the difference between wisdom and knowledge.

THE CHALLENGES

- Second-guessing what you believe to be true.
- Dealing with an excess of information may rev up your nervous system.

AFFIRMATIONS

- I know how to know.
- Options are to be explored.
- Curiosity leads to understanding.
- Being versatile yields opportunities.

SELF-CARE RITUALS

- Do breathing exercises.
- Research a wellness modality.

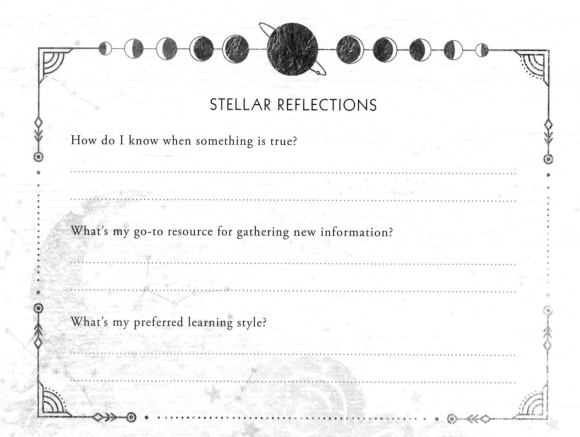

STELLAR REFLECTIONS

How do I know when something is true?

....

....

What's my go-to resource for gathering new information?

....

....

What's my preferred learning style?

....

....

Cancer Full Moon

THE OPPORTUNITIES

- Learning how to nourish yourself and others more efficiently.
- Making your workplace feel more homey.

THE CHALLENGES

- Emotionality may undermine authority.
- The need to attend to a flurry of responsibilities.

AFFIRMATIONS

- Being responsible nurtures me.
- I have a duty to protect myself.
- I trust my feelings.
- My roots are strong.

SELF-CARE RITUALS

- Clean out your pantry.
- Look through old photos.

STELLAR REFLECTIONS

Who, what, and where make me feel the most at home?

....

....

How can I further show my family how important my work is to me?

....

....

What gets in my way of sharing my needs with others?

....

....

Leo Full Moon

THE OPPORTUNITIES

- Adopting a childlike perspective can create a revolutionary solution.
- Seeing how being authentically yourself helps others.

THE CHALLENGES

- Being too self-focused may disrupt group dynamics.
- Pomp and circumstance obscure scientific facts.

AFFIRMATIONS

- It's important to make space for everyone.
- I contribute in a unique way.
- I love my inner child.
- I am creative.

SELF-CARE RITUALS

- Write a letter to your inner child.
- Give yourself a scalp massage.

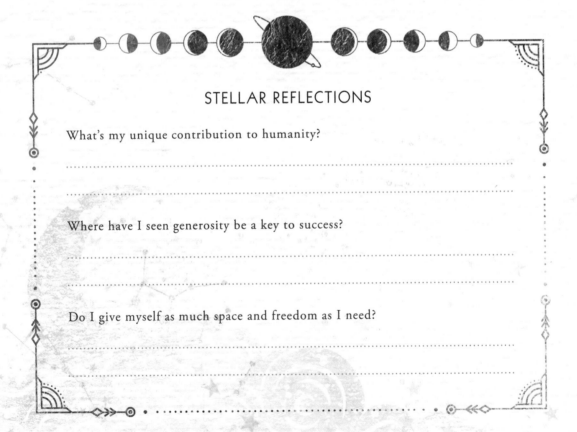

STELLAR REFLECTIONS

What's my unique contribution to humanity?

....

....

Where have I seen generosity be a key to success?

....

....

Do I give myself as much space and freedom as I need?

....

Virgo Full Moon

THE OPPORTUNITIES

- Perceiving how mind, body, and spirit are woven together leads to healing.

- Seeing the differences and the similarities.

THE CHALLENGES

- Confusing service with sacrifice.

- Perfectionism can lead to procrastination.

AFFIRMATIONS

- I am of service.

- Healing is my birthright.

- The parts make the whole.

- My perceptive skills are strong.

SELF-CARE RITUALS

- Decode a recent dream.

- Paint with watercolors.

STELLAR REFLECTIONS

In what ways am I drawn to be of service?

....

....

Does striving for perfection motivate me, set up a cycle of self-criticism, or both?

....

....

How can I better organize my days to create more ease?

....

....

Libra Full Moon

THE OPPORTUNITIES

- Forging alliances can help you pursue your desires.
- Using a diplomatic strategy aids in better championing an important cause.

THE CHALLENGES

- A propensity for compromise may stifle the pursuit of your aims.
- A partner's needs may cause you to feel overshadowed.

AFFIRMATIONS

- Justice ignites my soul.
- My value is strong.
- I am a good partner.
- I appreciate my own beauty.

SELF-CARE RITUALS

- Surround yourself with art.
- Hang out with a friend.

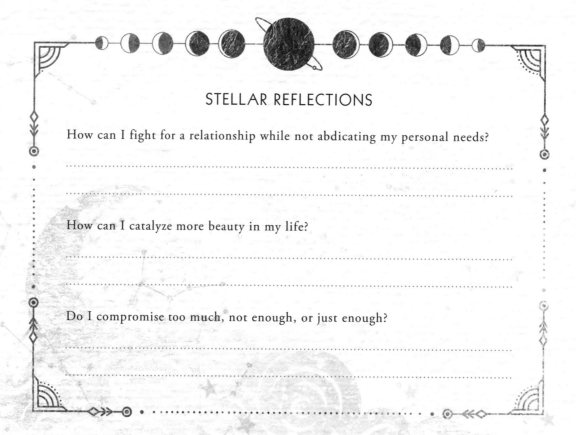

STELLAR REFLECTIONS

How can I fight for a relationship while not abdicating my personal needs?

....

....

How can I catalyze more beauty in my life?

....

....

Do I compromise too much, not enough, or just enough?

....

....

Scorpio Full Moon

THE OPPORTUNITIES

- Seeing how a tenacious approach helps override obstacles.

- Having a powerful sexual experience.

THE CHALLENGES

- Feeling torn between wanting change and wanting things to stay the same.

- Experiencing uncertainty about whether to take things at face value.

AFFIRMATIONS

- I trust my core instincts.

- Treasures reside below the surface.

- I own my power.

- I am resilient.

SELF-CARE RITUALS

- Read something erotic.

- Explore a mysterious subject.

STELLAR REFLECTIONS

In what ways would I describe myself as tenacious?

....

....

How has my sexuality evolved over the past few years?

....

....

How apt am I to dig below the surface when dealing with practical matters?

....

....

Sagittarius Full Moon

THE OPPORTUNITIES

- Stepping back allows you to see the bigger picture.
- Expanding your understanding of what's possible.

THE CHALLENGES

- A propensity to selectively use facts to push forth one's agenda.
- Nervous exhaustion caused by overstimulation.

AFFIRMATIONS

- I know how to know.
- Many things are possible.
- Discovery inspires me.
- I am hopeful.

SELF-CARE RITUALS

- Meditate by candlelight.
- Take a long walk.

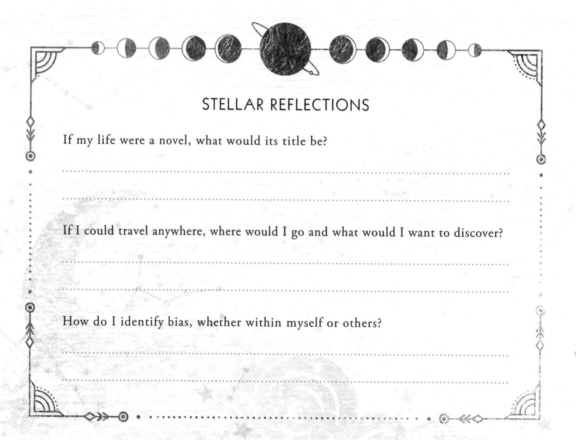

STELLAR REFLECTIONS

If my life were a novel, what would its title be?

....

....

If I could travel anywhere, where would I go and what would I want to discover?

....

....

How do I identify bias, whether within myself or others?

....

....

Capricorn Full Moon

THE OPPORTUNITIES

- Mastering the rules can yield a feeling of protection.
- Proceeding slowly feels very nourishing.

THE CHALLENGES

- Loyalties may be called into question.
- Uncertainty whether to take a direct or an indirect route.

AFFIRMATIONS

- I am responsible for my emotions.
- Time is on my side.
- My home nurtures me.
- I feel grounded.

SELF-CARE RITUALS

- Plan family activities.
- Read about your ancestry.

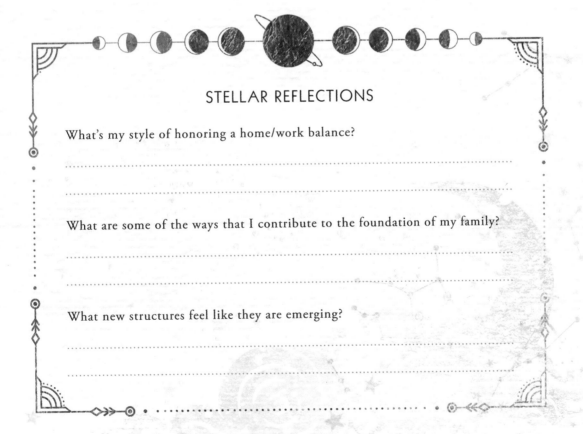

STELLAR REFLECTIONS

What's my style of honoring a home/work balance?

....

....

What are some of the ways that I contribute to the foundation of my family?

....

....

What new structures feel like they are emerging?

....

....

Aquarius Full Moon

THE OPPORTUNITIES

- Being inspired by art that promotes social causes.

- Discovering technology that connects you to your creativity.

THE CHALLENGES

- Tension between the needs of an organization and those of its members.

- An overly intellectual approach that limits creative expression.

AFFIRMATIONS

- I give voice to innovative solutions.

- I see the beauty of connections.

- The future is bright.

- I'm a creative thinker.

SELF-CARE RITUALS

- Participate in a group art project.

- Research health apps.

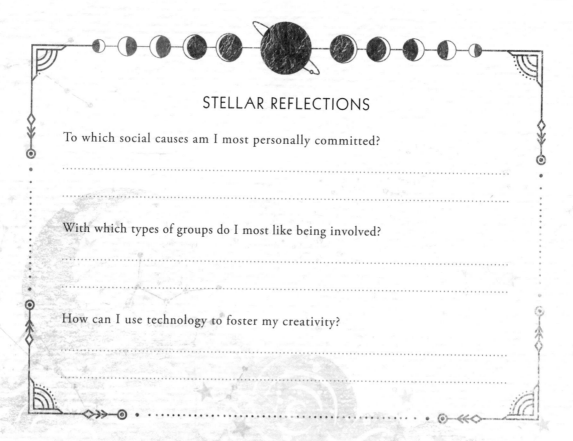

STELLAR REFLECTIONS

To which social causes am I most personally committed?

....

....

With which types of groups do I most like being involved?

....

....

How can I use technology to foster my creativity?

....

....

Pisces Full Moon

THE OPPORTUNITIES

- Learning new techniques to bolster your intuition.
- Realizing that forgiveness leads to healing.

THE CHALLENGES

- A wandering mind may have you miss some important details.
- Striving for perfection can derail progress.

AFFIRMATIONS

- I am love.
- My intuition is strong.
- Forgiveness heals.
- My dreams inspire me.

SELF-CARE RITUALS

- Take photographs.
- Forgive someone.

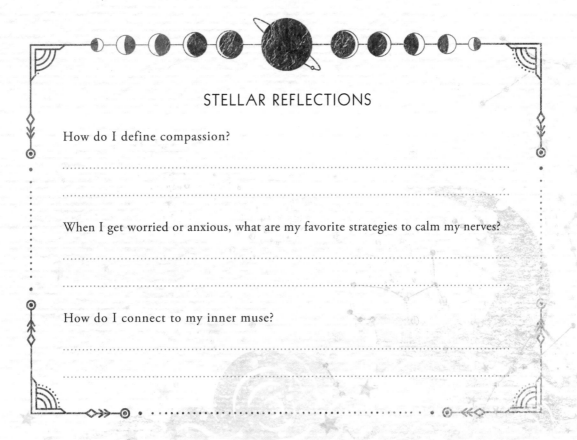

STELLAR REFLECTIONS

How do I define compassion?

....

....

When I get worried or anxious, what are my favorite strategies to calm my nerves?

....

....

How do I connect to my inner muse?

....

....

PART IV:

planetary retrogrades

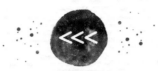

RETROGRADE BASICS

When a planet is in retrograde motion, it appears—from our perspective on Earth—to be traveling backward across the skyscape. Following the "as above, so below" axiom, just as the planets seem to be moving in a direction different than usual as they retrace their steps, so should we. This is the power of retrograde periods, notably those of the planets Mercury, Venus, and Mars. During these times we are given the invitation for do-overs, learning from the past and capturing new insights that can help us build a more complete understanding of ourselves and our place in the world.

Planetary retrogrades invite us to pause and slow down, and orient ourselves from a more internal and intuitive place. They are a time for reflection and heightened inner awareness. Instead of being exceptionally active in doing things, we may find ourselves more drawn toward just being. As we move more luxuriously, we may see things that we would have missed if we had kept on with our usual pace.

We revisit people, places, and situations in our lives; by doing so, we are gifted with gathering awareness that comes through reattending to arenas we have already experienced, getting to reexperience them through another lens. From this, we craft a more complete, and more holistic understanding from which springs more consciousness and empowerment. When it's a Mercury Retrograde, this understanding comes in the arenas of communication, education, and transport; with Venus, relationships, finances, and pleasure; and with Mars, pursuits, conflict resolution, and the nature of our desires.

Mercury, Venus, and Mars Retrograde periods have a bad reputation, with many people feeling that these times are harbingers of breakdowns and things going awry. Yet, if you align yourself with their planetary invitations, you can avoid stress and capitalize on the

Re-view Your Dreams

Dream incubation is a great self-care strategy to do during Mercury, Venus, and Mars Retrograde. A traditional practice with research studies bolstering its benefits, dream incubation involves asking your dreams to yield awareness about a particular topic in which you want further insights. Once you determine the focus of your query, you frame a simple and straight-forward question that acts as a prompt, encouraging your mind to hone in on the subject as you sleep. Write the question in your dream journal and then repeat it to yourself as you drift off to slumber. When you awaken, write down what you remember from your dream, then reflect upon it through the lens of your incubation intention.

opportunities they offer. One way to do this is to follow the *re-trograde strategy*, applying the prefix *re* to the activities that you undertake (such as re-write, re-evaluate, re-strategize, etc.). Experienced through this vantage point, you will begin to see how these periods can actually yield great benefit: the ability to perceive things you may not have previously seen, allowing you to refine your approach to life.

In the following sections, you'll discover perspectives and strategies that will help you make the most of Mercury, Venus, and Mars Retrograde. You'll also learn about self-care activities—including meditations, flower essences, and crystals—that can bolster your well-being as well as dreamwork intentions and Stellar Reflections journaling prompts to access new awareness.

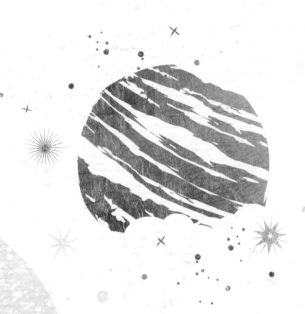

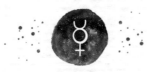

MERCURY RETROGRADE

In astrology, the planet Mercury governs communications, bridges, transportation, and the distribution of information and goods.

When Mercury is retrograde, we have the opportunity to revisit ideas from the past. In reexamining them, we can gain new insights that allow us to more clearly share our thoughts and move about in the world.

It's a time to go slowly and be exceptionally thoughtful about the delivery of information, goods, and services. Challenges can emerge if, instead of being patient, we hastily rush forward, whether in trying to understand something or in getting someone to understand our viewpoint. Doing so may limit our ability to access a slew of valuable information; it may also cause communication breakdowns and misunderstandings.

Mercury Retrograde is a period in which to focus upon unfinished business related to writing or design projects, understanding our transportation needs, assessing the tools we need to develop efficient communication, and re-attending to conversations that seem incomplete. It's an especially great time to do the following re-involved activities: re-write, re-edit, re-view, re-analyze, re-examine, re-calculate, and re-communicate.

The new perspective that can be accessed during Mercury Retrograde will help inform and strengthen your communication approaches, notably after this cycle is complete.

WHEN DOES IT OCCUR?

Mercury Retrograde lasts approximately three weeks and occurs three to four times a year. (Find a resource to discover Mercury Retrograde dates on page 252.)

OPPORTUNITIES FOR AWARENESS

Experiences we have during Mercury Retrograde may lead to:

- Finding new sources through which we can access information.
- Discovering alternative routes to get us to our chosen destination.
- Removing obstacles that restrict our communicating with ease.
- Better appreciating our unique learning style.
- Placing a greater value on our intuition.

STRATEGIES TO SIDESTEP STRESS

Minimize Mercury Retrograde challenges by employing these approaches:

- Ensure your tech devices and transport vehicles are in good working order.
- Finish your to-do list before attempting new projects.
- Be slow and thoughtful in communication.
- Double-check details of your travel itinerary.
- Have a back-up plan.

SELF-CARE SUGGESTIONS

Activities

- Re-read a favorite book.
- Take a break from social media.
- Try nondominant handwriting (see page 57 for more details).

Meditation: Breathing Meditation

As the respiratory system is under the guidance of Mercury, doing a meditation practice that focuses upon the breath may be especially aligned during this time. Find a comfortable sitting position that allows you to keep your spine straight. Relax your body. Close your eyes or gently gaze at something in front of you. Tune into your breath, noticing and following your inhalations and exhalations. Observe them, without attempting to adjust their pace; just breathe as you naturally do. Follow them with your mind's eye, paying attention to how your breath feels and where in your body you notice it moving through. If your mind wanders, don't judge yourself; just recognize that it drifted and bring your attention back to your breath. Start by doing this practice for five minutes a day, building up to twenty minutes or more.

Flower Essence: Cosmos

During Mercury Retrograde, we may access a flurry of information, both from the world around us as well as from our intuitive mind. It may feel challenging to synthesize all the insights we access and our minds may feel flooded and foggy, inhibiting our ability to clearly communicate. If you need a little assistance finding the words to readily express your ideas, thoughts, and feelings—and share them in an integrated way—consider Cosmos flower essence. (See page 20 for how to use flower essences.)

Crystal: Blue Lace Agate

One of the premier stones for communication, blue lace agate—a gem ruled by Mercury—is thought to nurture the throat chakra; it encourages a deeper connection to thoughts and feelings, as well as the confidence to express them. It's said to help people choose the words that will best get their point across. During Mercury Retrograde, hold the stone in your hand whenever you need support or place it on your nightstand or altar.

STELLAR REFLECTIONS

What do I need so that I can further trust my intuition?

....

....

Who from my past can help me solve a current problem I'm encountering?

....

....

How would I do over an important conversation that didn't go as planned?

....

....

Dreams of the Past

As retrograde periods are times when we retrace our steps, see whether the past plays a significant role in your dreams. This could manifest as the setting being one from a previous time in your life or even representing a historical period. Because we often run into or think about people from our past during Mercury, Venus, and Mars Retrograde, they may appear in your dreams in an even more concentrated way. If this happens, consider what they signify to you, whether related to how you view them or to the time in your life that they represent. Explore what their appearance in your dream may be offering you in terms of enhanced ways to share information (during Mercury Retrograde), deepen relationships (during Venus Retrograde), or pursue your aims (during Mars Retrograde).

WORKING WITH YOUR DREAMS

We can work with our dreams during Mercury Retrograde to access insights that can help us further understand how to strengthen our approach to communication.

Pay particular attention if symbols related to Mercury—including computers, books, mail, newspapers, transportation vehicles, bridges, siblings, messengers, and merchants—appear in your dreams. Reflect upon the images and see what they may be revealing to you. Given that our attention often returns to situations that occurred previously during retrograde periods, the past may also show up with more prevalence in your dreams (see left).

If you'd like to practice dream incubation (see page 238) during Mercury Retrograde, you can make inquiries to help you gain further insight into how to craft an important message, strengthen your relationships with your peers, and understand the way that your mind operates. For example, if you're working on a design project, you could ask your dream for creative solutions. If you've had a misunderstanding with a sibling, you could request clarity that will resolve the impasse. And if you're curious how to solve a problem that's been plaguing you, you can make that the focus of your dream incubation. While you can practice this any time during the retrograde cycle, you may find that it's more potent the days around the beginning and end of Mercury Retrograde.

VENUS RETROGRADE

In astrology, the planet Venus governs love, relationships, alliances, finances, beauty, pleasure, and things that have value.

When Venus is retrograde, we have the opportunity to reevaluate what we value. Relationships are one of the realms that are under heightened consideration during this time. Stumbling blocks that we experience with our partner, friends, or clients may be frustrating yet may also give us insight into ways we need to bolster our alliances. If aggravations arise, see what they reveal about the relationship, including whether you have realistic expectations for it. View this period as one in which you can gain greater awareness into how you approach partnerships and see whether you want to adjust the balance of the give and take that they feature.

As Venus Retrograde also gives us the opportunity to further understand the meaning of worth and richness, it's a time when we may learn great lessons regarding our finances. We can gain awareness about how we relate to and manage our money, as well as whether we feel we are fairly compensated for what we do. Additionally, we may find ourselves undertaking a cost/benefit analysis that helps us further understand whether the price we pay for things is commensurate with the value that we derive from them.

People, perspectives, and places from your past may provide you with great treasures that help you access one of the big lessons of this time—ways to bolster a deeper understanding of just how valuable you truly are.

WHEN DOES IT OCCUR?

Venus Retrograde lasts approximately six weeks and occurs about every eighteen months. (Find a resource to discover Venus Retrograde dates on page 252.)

OPPORTUNITIES FOR AWARENESS

Experiences we have during Venus Retrograde may lead to:

- Further understanding what brings us pleasure.
- Discovering ways relationships can offer us more reward.
- Better understanding what love means.
- Honing our ability to manage our finances.
- Learning to be a better negotiator.

STRATEGIES TO SIDESTEP STRESS

Minimize Venus Retrograde challenges by employing these approaches:

- Don't rush to conclusions regarding a relationship.
- Watch your potential to romanticize someone or something.
- Value your unique skills and talents.
- Be mindful of how much you compromise.
- Consciously consider whether something has true value.

SELF-CARE SUGGESTIONS

Activities

- Reach out to a friend you haven't spoken to in a while.
- Take a look at your finances.
- Give yourself a facial.

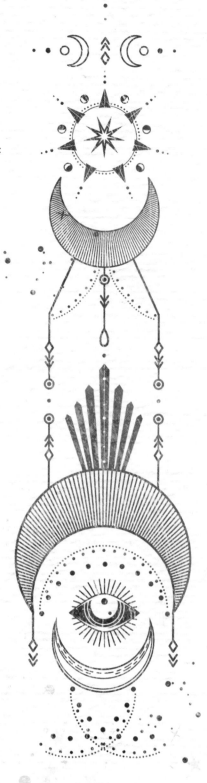

Meditation: Tonglen Meditation

Since relationships are a central focus during Venus Retrograde, Tonglen meditation—which involves holding others with compassion—seems like an especially aligned practice to do during this time. Finding a comfortable spot to sit, relax your body. Consider someone you know who is suffering and whom you want to help. As you inhale, imagine you are breathing in their pain (you can even visualize that you're breathing in heaviness or darkness). As you exhale, breathe out compassion and healing, sending it to them. Do this practice for five minutes to start, building up to twenty minutes. Tonglen need not be restricted to a formal meditation practice; any time you see someone suffering, you can take a moment to breathe in their sorrow and breathe out caring and tenderhearted feelings. Steeped in the action of compassion, Tonglen may be transformative for you as well as the relationship.

Flower Essence: Buttercup

Venus Retrograde offers us the opportunity to more fully appreciate and value ourselves, owning our uniqueness and embracing our self-worth. As this is the support that the flower essence Buttercup provides, it can be a wonderful elixir for this time. It helps us connect to our inner radiant light and shift a propensity for self-doubt into self-appreciation. It's an especially good remedy to help us embrace the richness of who we are in times when we are apt to judge ourselves by external markers of success. (See page 20 for how to use flower essences.)

Crystal: Rose Quartz

Rose quartz inspires love of all types—including that which we give ourselves—and helps us open to more kindness, tenderness, and understanding. It invokes joy and peace, elevates self-worth, and enhances our affinity to beauty. Known as the "love stone," rose quartz is often the crystal people work with to deepen their relationships. It is said to nurture the heart chakra, the energy center that's thought to connect us to our ability to embrace love and compassion. During Venus Retrograde, place rose quartz on your altar or nightstand, set it on your heart during meditation, or use a face roller made from this gemstone as part of your skin-care regimen.

WORKING WITH YOUR DREAMS

We can work with our dreams during Venus Retrograde to access awareness to help clarify what we value, determine what shifts we may want to make in our relationships, and discover how to bring more beauty and pleasure into our lives.

Pay particular attention if symbols related to Venus—including lovers, luxury items, money, mirrors, artwork, objects of beauty, and cosmetics—appear in your dreams. Reflect upon the images and see what they may be revealing to you. Given that retrogrades often have us reviewing situations that came before, images of the past may be a common feature of your dreams (see page 242).

STELLAR REFLECTIONS

How do I define beauty?

....

....

....

What gets in the way of my valuing myself?

....

....

....

What really fulfills me in a relationship?

....

....

....

If you'd like to practice dream incubation (see page 238) during Venus Retrograde, you can craft inquiries to gain further insight into relationship dynamics, how to proceed with a creative project, or find a solution to a financial matter. For example, if you're faced with a partnership predicament, you could ask for resolution strategies. If you're looking for new income streams, you could beckon your dream to provide you with ideas. And if you're uncertain whether to proceed with a big purchase, you can make that the focus of your incubation inquiry. While you can practice this any time during the retrograde cycle, you may find that it's more potent the days around the beginning and end of Venus Retrograde.

Tonglen Meditation

A style of meditation rooted in Tibetan Buddhism, *tonglen* means "sending and receiving." This reflects the focus of this contemplative practice in which you direct compassion and healing to those whom you hold in your mind's eye. With roots back to the 10th century CE, tonglen meditation has become more popular recently owing to current-day Buddhist scholars and practitioners including Pema Chodron.

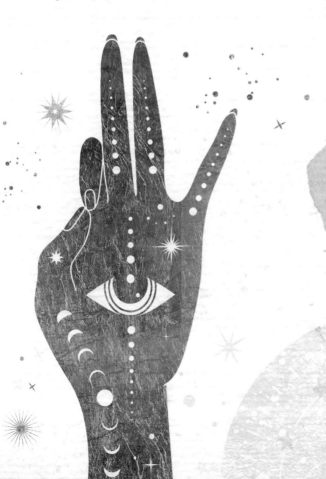

MARS RETROGRADE

In astrology, the planet Mars governs willpower, energy, passion, anger, desire, battlefields, and the urge to fight and champion.

When Mars is retrograde, we have the opportunity to discover new strategies that will help us meet our aims. It's a time in which we are rewarded with awareness by going slow and taking pauses when necessary. Instead of carrying on at the same speed we're used to, we can recognize a more optimal and sustainable pace. These months offer us great insights into the arsenal of tools we have at our disposal and which ones may better help us get the job done.

That said, Mars Retrograde can yield frustrations that emerge from setbacks and postponements; after all, Mars reflects an energy that likes to move forward, while retrograde periods are ones in which we're encouraged to go back and retrace already visited territory. Watch for excess anger that can be stoked if you don't get what you want when you want it.

We may become upset if gratification is delayed, or we can't propel ourselves with the momentum to which we're accustomed. Impatience may rage and lead to mishaps if we're not careful. Be aware of the potential for irritation or inflammation, whether experienced in your mind or in your body.

By re-evaluating actions we've taken in the past, as well as further understanding our relationship with anger, we may find ourselves discovering new solutions that can lead to more sustainable progress after the retrograde period is complete.

WHEN DOES IT OCCUR?

Mars Retrograde lasts roughly ten weeks and occurs about every twenty-six months. (Find a resource to discover Mars Retrograde dates on page 252.)

OPPORTUNITIES FOR AWARENESS

Experiences we have during Mars Retrograde may lead to:

- Clarifying just what it is that we desire.
- Understanding our hidden motivations.
- Seeing how to more efficiently use our energy.
- Relating more consciously to our anger.
- Becoming better at handling conflict.

STRATEGIES TO SIDESTEP STRESS

Minimize Mars Retrograde challenges by employing these approaches:

- Avoid shortcuts.
- Watch out for bouts of impatience.
- Be aware of the impact of having a very short fuse.
- Move as slowly and mindfully as possible.
- Determine the optimal time to air a grievance.

SELF-CARE SUGGESTIONS

Activities
- Do a few gentle stretches during your morning routine.
- Learn some self-defense moves.
- End your shower with a blast of cold water.

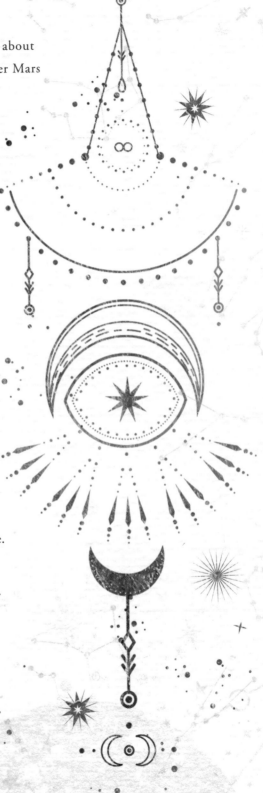

Meditation: Walking Meditation

Since Mars Retrograde is a time to tap into the wisdom of conscious movement, walking meditation may be a powerful way to connect to greater relaxation and awareness. Stand still for a few moments, feeling grounded in your body as you concentrate on your breath. Begin walking slowly and deliberately, being mindful of your steps. Turn your attention to the sensations you're experiencing, whether your breath, the feeling of your body moving, the connection between your feet and the ground, the ambient noises you hear, or whatever sights your eyes take in. If your mind wanders, just come back to noticing the sensations. Begin doing this practice for five minutes, building up to twenty minutes or more. You can practice this outdoors or choose a path in your home in which you can walk back and forth.

Flower Essence: Blackberry

Mars Retrograde provides us with a stellar opportunity to learn more about our willpower and how to strengthen it. We can discover how to marry our ideas and desires, tapping into the energy necessary to work on behalf of manifesting our goals. This is the realm of Blackberry flower essence, which can help us unearth the wealth of our will so we can take more conscious and decisive action. (See page 20 for how to use flower essences.)

Crystal: Garnet

Like Mars, garnet is aligned with champions; it is traditionally known as a warrior stone, used to inspire protection and courage. It has invigorating properties, thought to help support the flow of *chi* (life force energy) and shield against negative environmental influences. Garnet is also used for helping people connect to their passion and libido and is said to help balance the sex drive. During Mars Retrograde, carry garnet with you as a shield of protection and source of strength.

WORKING WITH YOUR DREAMS

We can work with our dreams during Mars Retrograde to further understand how to resolve conflict, connect to our desires, and fight for what we truly want.

Pay particular attention if symbols related to Mars appear in your dreams; these may include fire, battles, knives, weapons, warriors, sharp objects, sexual pursuits, and the color red. Reflect upon the images and see what they may be revealing to you. Since

STELLAR REFLECTIONS

What's my usual response when I'm confronted with fear: fight, flight, or freeze?

....

....

What's my relationship with anger?

....

....

What is it that I truly desire?

....

....

retrograde periods have us turning to things that occurred prior, situations from the past may arise more readily in our dreams during this time (see page 242 for more).

If you'd like to practice dream incubation (see page 238) during Mars Retrograde, you can craft inquiries that can help you gain further insight into how to connect to your resolve, tap into your sexuality, or pursue an aim important to you. For example, if you're struggling with accessing your erotic nature, you could ask your dream to provide insights. If you want to discover a breakthrough to a conflict you're having, you could frame your inquiry around that. And if you're wondering how to safeguard and defend something that's important to you, you may want to turn your dream incubation attention to that discovery. While you can practice this any time during the retrograde cycle, you may find that it's more potent the days around the beginning and end of Mars Retrograde.

resources

Cast your chart and discover your Sun, Moon, and Ascendant signs at astro.com or by consulting with a professional astrologer. Find information to help you identify when you're experiencing one of the Stellar Life Stages at StephanieGailing.com. There you can also find dates for upcoming New and Full Moons as well as the retrograde cycles of Mercury, Venus, and Mars.

....

There are a vast array of books available through which you can learn about astrology and self-care topics. Here are a few of my favorites:

ASTROLOGY

Arroyo, Stephen. *Astrology, Karma, and Transformation*, 2nd Ed. CRCS Publications, 1992

Cornell, Howard Leslie. *Encyclopedia of Medical Astrology*. Echo Point Books & Media, 2017

Greene, Liz. *The Luminaries*. Red Wheel / Weiser, 1992

Hand, Robert. *Horoscope Symbols*. Schiffer Pub Ltd, 1981

Hickey, Isabel M. *Astrology: A Cosmic Science*, 4th Ed. CRCS Publications, 2011

Hillman, Laurence. *Planets in Play*. Tarcher, 2007

Jansky, Robert Carl. *Astrology, Nutrition and Health*. Schiffer Pub Ltd, 1971

Nicholas, Chani. *You Were Born for This*. HarperOne, 2020

Ridder-Patrick, Jane. *A Handbook of Medical Astrology*. CrabApple Press, 2006

Starck, Marcia. *Healing with Astrology*. Crossing Press, 1997

SELF-CARE

Gailing, Stephanie. *The Complete Book of Dreams*. Wellfleet Press, 2020

Gerber, Richard. *Vibrational Medicine*, 3rd Ed. Bear & Company, 2001

Kaminiski, Patricia, and Katz, Richard. *Flower Essence Repertory*. Flower Essence Services, 2004

Meza, Melina. *The Art of Sequencing*, Volume 1. Melina Meza Press, 2007

Mojay, Gabriel. *Aromatherapy for Healing the Spirit*. Healing Arts Press, 2000

Pitchford, Paul. *Healing with Whole Foods*. North Atlantic Books, 1993

Ryman, Daniele. *The Aromatherapy Bible*. Piatkus Books, 2002

Scheffer, Mechthild. *The Encyclopedia of Bach Flower Therapy*. Healing Arts Press, 2001

acknowledgments

The Complete Guide to Astrological Self-Care has been a labor of love, one that would not have come to life were it not for so many special people:

John Foster, editor extraordinaire, whose championing of my work and confidence in me as a writer are gifts that I will always treasure. The amazing team at Wellfleet Press—including Rage Kindelsperger, Laura Drew, Cara Donaldson, and Lydia Anderson—for creating this book and sharing it with the world, and Sosha Davis and Kate Smith for making it so beautiful. My husband Sebastiano and my dear family and friends for their unending support. My grandfather Abe who always encouraged me to be an author. Aimee Hartstein, for our shared love of astrology, and Heidi Lender, for always knowing wellness astrology was my path. Simone, Ben, and Margot, who inspire me to make this world a better place. Melina Meza, for her invaluable contributions to the yoga poses sections. Ingrid Emerick and Laurie Baum who many years ago helped me bring this book's vision to life. And finally, to all the astrologers and health-care practitioners, past and present, whose contributions to the healing arts enable us to more readily pursue a life of stellar well-being.

about the author

Stephanie Gailing is a life guide, wellness astrologer, and author with more than twenty-five years of experience. Her unique approach to healing weaves together compassion-based coaching, self-care strategies, dreamwork, and astrological insights. In addition to working directly with individuals, couples, and organizations throughout the world, Stephanie regularly teaches workshops and writes about holistic well-being. Co-host of the *So Divine!* podcast, Stephanie is the author of *The Complete Book of Dreams*. She holds a Certificate in EcoPsychology from Pacifica University, an Advanced Diploma in Coaching from New York University, and an MS in Nutrition from Bastyr University. You can find more about her work at StephanieGailing.com.

index